04/29/14

Praise for *Whole Health*

"The underlying premise of *Whole Health* embodies concepts of energy in healing that are at once ancient and futuristic. Such concepts lead us all to an integrative, holistic, and evolutionary paradigm of healing that differs profoundly and refreshingly from the reductionistic biomedical worldview of conventional medicine today. Read this book and introduce yourself to the future of medicine, available to you right now."

> —Dana Ullman, M.P.H., C.C.H., coauthor of Everybody's Guide to Homeopathic Medicine and contributing writer to The Huffington Post

"*Whole Health* is loaded with many gems about health and wholeness. I highly recommend it."

> —Christiane Northrup, M.D., ob-gyn physician and author of the New York Times bestsellers Women's Bodies, Women's Wisdom and The Wisdom of Menopause

"Mark Mincolla unearths and shares a treasure chest of healing potential in his instant classic *Whole Health*. This is a must-read for all those searching for ways to increase their ability to take control of their nutritional, emotional, and physical well-being."

> —Keith Ablow, M.D., psychiatrist, New York Times–bestselling author of Inside the Mind of Scott Peterson and coauthor of The 7, and member of Fox News's "Medical A-Team"

"*Whole Health* has a wealth of information about how to assess an individual's state of health, and how to use energy and nutrition to achieve physical, mental, emotional, and spiritual balance. It will undoubtedly prove of great value to all those interested in improving their own health, and to health care practitioners wishing to increase their knowledge and understanding to provide even better care for their patients."

> —Penelope Quest, M.Sc., B.A., author of Reiki for Life

WHOLE
HEALTH

WHOLE
HEALTH

*A Holistic Approach
to Healing for the 21st Century*

MARK MINCOLLA, PH.D.

JEREMY P. TARCHER / PENGUIN

a member of Penguin Group (USA)

New York

JEREMY P. TARCHER/PENGUIN
Published by the Penguin Group
Penguin Group (USA) LLC
375 Hudson Street
New York, New York 10014

penguin.com
A Penguin Random House Company

Most Tarcher/Penguin books are available at special quantity discounts
for bulk purchase for sales promotions, premiums, fund-raising, and educational needs.
Special books or book excerpts also can be created to fit specific needs.
For details, write: Special.Markets@us.penguingroup.com.

Library of Congress Cataloging-in-Publication Data
Mincolla, Mark Dana.
Whole health : a holistic approach to healing for the 21st century /
Mark Mincolla, Ph.D.
p.   cm.
ISBN 978-0-399-16501-6
1. Health—Popular works.   2. Mental healing—Popular works.
3. Holistic medicine.   I. Title.
RA776.5.M533   2013   2013036565
613—dc23

Printed in the United States of America
1   3   5   7   9   10   8   6   4   2

Book design by Tanya Maiboroda

I would like to dedicate

Whole Health

to my grandson Elijah.

Your miracles await you from deep within.

CONTENTS

FOREWORD
by Bernie Siegel, M.D.

In *Whole Health*, Mark Mincolla has put together a book of great value. This book offers us information that can make a difference in our lives and health. I also know, however, that without inspiration, the information will be ignored. Mark and I both want you to know that we care about you, and if you had an abusive past and did not feel loved, you can abandon your past and let us help to re-parent you and to help you to find self-love and the health benefits that come with it.

What Mark shares, he has learned from his experiences and not the preconceived beliefs that would only serve to interfere with the healing process. True healing demands that the face of medicine be changed. Rather than simply be provided a diagnosis and prescription, the patient needs to be empowered with the preventive wisdom to help avoid future illnesses. Medicine also needs to educate its physicians to focus on treating the patient's total experience and to not ignore the factors that led to their illness.

We also need to learn, as Mark has, from patients who do well. It drives me crazy when doctors say to patients who are doing well, "You're doing very well. Whatever it is you are doing, keep it up." What they need to say is, "You are doing very well. Tell me what you are doing." We can all learn from success by not calling it spontaneous or miraculous but by seeing that healing can be self-induced, and that our lifestyle and nutrition can be our medicine. We all have the potential to heal but have to be willing to do the work to allow it to happen. Our body needs to know we love it; then our entire life will get the message and will do all it can to help us heal and grow in a transformational way. We need to treat the whole picture and be truly holistic.

The word *doctor* derives its meaning from "teacher." We practitioners need to be more like coaches who criticize in a constructive way so that our patients become healthier and better performers, but our players will have to show up for practice if we are going to see any results. We care about you and want you to know that you are worthy of compassion and love no matter how painful your past experience was with the authority figures in your life.

When you lose your health, we'll be here to help you find it. You must go beyond viewing the process of disease as punishment, or wellness as something you deserve. I want you to take as good care of yourself as you do your beloved pets. When we love our lives and bodies, our internal chemistry helps us to heal and grow in a transformational way. True wellness is not about trying to avoid death but about healing our lives and bodies and benefiting from the health that comes with it.

A study of Harvard students published in *Nature* in 1998 showed that only one-fourth of those who felt loved by their parents suffered a major illness by midlife, while almost 100 percent of those who did not feel loved by their parents had suffered a major illness in the same time span.

Our lives are stored in our bodies, and if we do not respond to what is within us, someday the body will present us with the bill. Mark's work can help you to find self-empowerment and free yourself from unhealthy addictions and behaviors.

Medicine is limited by its beliefs and what it is willing to accept and research. If it can't explain something, it rejects it. We need to open our minds and beliefs, and Mark can help us to find the way to true healing and health. When I first decided to open my mind and my beliefs, I was criticized and rejected because what I wanted to research wasn't believed and accepted by the medical establishment. Decades later, the work is now getting done because beliefs have changed. Mind, body, and spirit are a unit, not separate entities, and they need to be treated as such.

We need to understand that when we wage war against disease, we empower the enemy. When we seek to find peace and heal, the disease is eliminated in the healing process. The ability to heal is built into all living things. Bacteria alter their genes and resist antibiotics. We cut our finger and don't bleed to death. The key issue in our vulnerability is to understand that our emotions create our internal chemistry, and can help us to resist or be vulnerable to disease. We need to pay attention to what is killing us and not just what symptoms we are complaining about. When we lose our health, we need to simply look for it. It's important that we don't see disease as a punishment, or health as something we deserve.

The medical profession needs to learn from Mark by not just prescribing pills but empowering patients and treating their experience. Doctors also need to accept criticism and let their patients become their teachers too. Tourists do not understand what natives are going through and experiencing. I try to help people to learn how to stop being good patients, or submissive sufferers, and become "respants," or responsible participants. Doctors need to define why some patients do better, learn from them, and help all patients to incorporate those traits into their lives and personalities, as Mark has done.

When people make the "right" choices for themselves, whether it means eating vegetables or undergoing medical treatments, they become empowered. When we love the child within us and understand true health, change will occur. When we see the world through a grandmother's eyes and not the eyes of a CEO, good health will bloom and blossom accordingly. I was born an ugly duckling, but had a grandmother who massaged and loved me, so those healing memories still remain within my body.

We are all unique, yet we have certain things in common, and Mark treats the things that deplete our energy and our ability to heal. Someday life force, consciousness, and energy will be scientific and incorporated into medicine and healing. I know from experience what we are capable of accomplishing when we direct our life force the way wires carry energy from a battery. When this is all accepted, mind-body-spirit will all be understood as one, and food will be seen as a source of energy that keeps us well, not just a medication.

The way to accomplish change is to rehearse and practice becoming the person you want to be. Mark's work can help train and coach you in this process. As I have said, our lives are stored within us, and if the wounds are not healed, the body will one day present us with its bill. We need to understand that while there is such a thing as survival behavior, we can choose to be empowered to change with the help of people like Mark Mincolla, and *Whole Health*.

INTRODUCTION

Day in, day out—over the past thirty years—tens of thousands of people have found their way to me in search of alternative health care strategies to ameliorate their troubling symptoms. They continue to routinely present with symptoms of cancer, heart disease, multiple sclerosis, rheumatoid arthritis, lupus, asthma, psoriasis, cirrhosis, irritable bowel syndrome . . . the list is never ending. Happily, and curiously, I can report that many of them successfully reverse their symptoms and go on to experience remarkable recoveries. Their recoveries have nothing to do with any fad diets or miracle pills. They are the result of a natural, alternative health care system that I've developed over the past three decades, which I call the Whole Health Healing System.

The Whole Health Healing System integrates elements of classical Chinese medicine, personalized nutrition, and extrasensory energy medicine. It is a system that inspires, empowers, and teaches its patients and students how to attain balance in body, mind, and spirit. One of the principal aims of this time-tested healing system is to teach patients that everything is energy, and that by learning to balance their vital energies with the proper corresponding food energies, they can prevent the onset of many inflammatory symptoms associated with their presenting diagnosis. They are energetically tested for food intolerances and instructed to avoid the foods that fail their bodies. The results have been nothing short of miraculous. In fact, I've found this "addition through subtraction" strategy to be so consistently effective at eliminating symptoms that it begs some very important questions.

What is disease? Do most of the patients whom I routinely help really have what they were diagnosed with? Does today's medical community truly understand what disease is? Or has disease simply become a host of symptoms named and classified to fit the prevailing pharmaceutical models of treatment?

The medical establishment has traditionally thought of disease as an abnormal condition, often triggered by external factors, causing pain, suffering, and/or the death of an organism. The medical orthodoxy appears to be completely unaware of the fact that food intolerances have become causal root factors masquerading as disease, as they are now responsible for triggering many disease symptoms. Disease begins with a breach of homeostasis. When any organism becomes imbalanced in body, mind, and/or spirit, disease is the inevitable, natural result.

In my world, homeostasis is most often breached by the inflammatory toxicity of food. Our genetically modified, pesticide-, saturated fat–, and trans fat–riddled, irradiated, sugary, fermented foods are making us sick. In fact, I believe that our denatured diet is making us so sick that its side effects are now mimicking, contributing to, and/or causing many of the great diseases of our time. When no more dairy results in no more asthma, then asthma isn't really asthma—it's a toxic-food intolerance. When no more gluten results in no more eczema, then eczema isn't eczema—it's a toxic-food intolerance. When no more saturated fats results in no more heart disease, then heart disease isn't heart disease—it's a toxic-food intolerance. When no more sugar and fermentation result in no more cancer, then cancer isn't cancer—it's a toxic-food intolerance.

Rather than simply subtracting the causal root of the symptoms, the current medical model insists on assigning symptoms a formal disease name so that they can match them up with a pharmaceutical strategy to treat the symptoms.

We've all had a good laugh at the *National Lampoon*–like pharmaceutical television commercials: "May cause dizziness, racing heart, insomnia, confusion, bladder/bowel irritation, lower back pain, urinary frequency, night sweats, nausea, a sudden drop in blood pressure, and in some cases death." According to Melody Petersen, author of *Our Daily Meds*, 100,000 Americans are killed by prescription drugs each year. That's 270 deaths every day! More than twice the number of people killed in car crashes. This staggering number of deaths doesn't even include those due to medical error, clearly revealing the potential dangers of pharmaceutical medications. In spite of these cold, hard facts, 65 percent of Americans continue to take prescription drugs, at a cost of $250 billion per year. Food and medicine are fast becoming the new diseases.

The medical orthodoxy will always have a place in our lives, but its role is clearly diminishing. We are in the midst of great change, where people are beginning to take a more active role in their own health care. The treatment of disease has become unaffordable on a myriad of levels and the world is rapidly turning to new models of disease prevention. Moreover, people the world over are rapidly outgrowing the mechanisms espoused by the current Western practice of medicine.

The present transformation is generating a great paradigm shift, not just in medicine but in consciousness. Moving forward, we will continue to see greater patient demand for health care treatment that evokes higher awareness. By now, we all know that when our body aches, so too does our spirit. We also know that much of what lies at the root of our ailing spirit is a broken heart.

We have outgrown the coldhearted mechanism of modern medicine, and our tolerance of pharmaceutical greed is at last wearing thin. We are multidimensional, energetic beings with an increasing desire to know more of our own greater depths. Our medicines merely keep us alive. Our need is for healing wisdoms that show us the way to a more whole and healthy life.

There is a growing hunger to go deeper and to know life beyond the material level. Our changing world is in the midst of a learning curve of epic proportions. The world's destiny to discover its true wholeness has at last arrived. The Whole Health Healing System was designed to assist in this great discovery.

CHAPTER 1

EVERYTHING IS ENERGY

A NEW CYCLE

Everything is energy, and energy is in a constant state of flux. While you and I have been conditioned and inculcated to believe in a material-based reality, quantum mechanics has proven that we and everything that appears to us as matter are in fact, comprised of 99.999 percent energy and only 0.001 percent matter. This concept, once relevant perhaps only to physics aficionados and academics, has suddenly found its way into the collective consciousness. We are all slowly getting used to the idea that we are energy and, as with all energy, we are constantly changing. Even now, our present rate of change is accelerating at an increasingly rapid pace.

In 2011, the Nobel Prize in Physics was awarded to Saul Perlmutter, Adam G. Riess, and Brian P. Schmidt, for their 1998 discovery of the universe's accelerated expansion. When we say that the universe is expanding at an accelerated rate, the underlying acknowledgment is that all the energy that makes up the universe is also expanding at an accelerated rate.

You and I are what make up the universe. Our subtlest conscious/unconscious, positive/negative thoughts, and emotional energies are exponentially accelerating. As our consciousness and unconsciousness both expand, you and I have the opportunity to cultivate our own unique potential to manifest more powerfully than ever before. Our thought energies have always preceded our ability to create, but never have they had such force behind them. Accelerated universal expansion hasn't just added fuel to our positive thought energy—it has empowered our negative thought energies as well.

With everything speeding up, our thinking is more prone to impulse, and our negative unconscious thoughts are manifesting as disease with far greater force. We must not underestimate the effects that these changes impose on our health. We need to be very clear about the fact that we are gaining an increase in thought power over the well-being and destiny of our own lives. During this time of great change, it is essential that we emphasize the importance of cultivating a higher consciousness to preside over our thoughts and emotions. More than ever, the manifest power of our thoughts and emotions has the potential to heal disease, but we must also keep in mind that these same thoughts and emotions can also create disease. We are at a tipping point of epic proportions, and the transformation we are now facing is also shifting the framework and values of our entire social structure.

The crushing blow of such a dramatic shift is creating a need for alternative support systems. Natural healing, spiritual enlightenment, personal development, and self-empowerment systems are beginning to be formalized and become more mainstream. These systems are representative of a new generation of cultural models that are no longer centered on administrative power. Instead they are focused on the education and empowerment of the individual.

The Whole Health Healing System represents a radical change in health care consciousness—a departure from the material toward an extrasensory and energy-based approach to health care. It is but one small change driven by the wheels of a much greater cycle of transformation. A consciousness revolution that reaches beyond the boundaries of time, space, and dimension has opened doors to new vistas of possibility, liberating us from the former constraints of material limitation. Our perception of reality will be forever changed, as a powerful new multiverse cycle (i.e., a cycle recognizing the infinite number of universes) is realized.

Within this new cycle, the seeds of a cultural revolution are being sown, as we bear witness to the germination of a future where our ability to heal reaches far beyond matter and into the realm of energy. Many are intuiting new wisdoms that reveal our power to effectively channel healing with intention alone, irrespective of time, space, or dimension. By integrating healing arts from our ancestral pasts with our own untapped powers, we are crafting new systems of medicine that are being mastered by laypersons around the world.

The power of the pharmaceutical pill will be equaled—if not surpassed—by the personal powers of consciousness, belief, and intention. As we continue to move through this changing multiversal cycle, we will soon come to realize that we have always possessed these powers to heal. The realization of such personal power will be met with both great anticipation and resistance, for the prospect of such radical change has the capacity to both excite and frighten.

Changing multiversal cycles trigger radical paradigm shifts in the world. A paradigm shift is described as a radical change in the theoretical framework of life. More to the point, paradigm shifts drastically alter those realities accepted as cultural norms, but then, cultural norms are largely based on mutable foundations such as mass perception (or belief through repetition), technology, inculcation, and economics.

Perception is a reflection of that which a given culture believes it's observing. Technology expands the baseline of what is observable. Inculcation is the cognitive downloading that establishes and sanctions belief norms. Economic factors reinforce cultural belief by generating a system of reward around it.

Imagine if we had a full-scale visit by a technologically advanced culture of extraterrestrials. Our reality perception would experience an immediate shock. Our most advanced technologies would suddenly become obsolete. Our petroleum- and motor-driven industries would seem antiquated overnight. Our inculcation processes would be thrown into a state of disarray, and our economic structures would crash until they could adapt. Sound a little far-fetched? It's happened many times before.

After thousands of years of uninterrupted natural living, Native Americans had their once "dreamlike" reality shock-shifted into just such a sudden nightmare by the arrival of the first European settlers. Their once foundational perceptions of reality, technology, inculcation, and economic structure were swiftly obliterated by the invading alien culture.

More recently, our culture has experienced radical reality shifts in the social sciences, psychology, marketing, and technology. In 1931, Konrad Zuse sparked a radical shift with his advent of the first freely programmable computer. Thousands of years of molecular brain technology were suddenly jolted by nanotechnology. In addition, we have undergone radical transitions from Ptolemaic to Copernican cosmology, from biogenesis to spontaneous generation, and from behaviorist to cognitive approaches in psychology.

Change is constant, and radical paradigm shifts are the most drastic forms of change that alter reality. But perhaps the greatest of all paradigm shifts is the one taking place in all of our lives as we speak. The very foundations of material reality we've been programmed to see and believe are vanishing right before our eyes.

Quantum mechanics represents a game changer that may have taken more than a century to embed itself into the mass consciousness, but make no mistake about it, quantum mechanics is making its presence known. This shift away from a mechanistic to a quantum reality is said to have begun as far back as 1857, with Gustav Kirchhoff's theory of "black body" radiation. Following more than 150 years of contributions from the likes of Einstein, Heisenberg, Maxwell, and Bohr, quantum mechanics has at last begun to creep into the collective psyche.

Quantum is Latin for "how much." A quantum of energy refers to a specific amount of energy that is proportional to frequency. The traditional biological sciences are based on a material-based reality. With quantum mechanics, however, reality is based on frequencies of energy. After thousands of years of material illusion, we have begun to understand that reality always was and forever will be energy-based.

Not unlike all material appearances, we, too, are energy. Our glands, organs, tissues, and cells are but vibrating particles of energy. In fact, all human anatomical frequencies have been precisely measured for their energy frequencies:

Bone: 38–43 MHz (megahertz—millions of cycles per second)
Heart: 67–70 Hz (hertz—cycles per second)
Thymus: 65–68 Hz
Thyroid: 62–68 Hz
Pancreas: 60–80 Hz
Lungs: 58–65 Hz
Liver: 55–60 Hz
Brain: 4–30 Hz

Everything within us and everywhere around us is a vibrating sea of energy that generates fields—and fields create the appearance of form. From subatomic particles to atoms, molecules, DNA, cells, tissues, organs, organisms, planets, galaxies, the universe, the multiverse, and the cosmos—everything is energy.

Everything in our world is made up of unseen energy that gives the appearance of matter. Objects that appear solid, such as animals, plants, trees, droplets of rain, and stars, are all composed of energy. Matter describes the physical appearance of all things, while energy represents their flowing action. I like to think of water as a metaphor for energy and ice as a metaphor for the appearance of matter. Reality, as we in the modern West have come to know it, has always been centered on the "ice cubes," but we're beginning to take note of the "water" that makes the cubes of life appear to be solid.

It's really not so much about what we're looking at. It's more about what we've been taught to see. Cultural programming determines what people believe they see. Every culture requires cognitive foundations from which it establishes its belief systems. Structures must be put in place to support the foundation of accepted cultural reality before the masses can be expected to embrace them. For example, whereas we in the West have been programmed to see and believe in a material reality, the Eastern world understands and embraces energy-based reality. Our respective cultural programming has been set up to support what we believe in and, though deeply rooted in our way of life, it is far from fixed. What you and I have been taught to accept as reality is the result of cognitive downloading. Unfortunately, our downloading is flimsy, at best.

Before beginning your day, think about the energetic aspects of the apparent material life you're living. Take a moment to focus your attention on yourself and everything around you from an energetic standpoint rather than a material perspective. As you walk down the hallway to the bathroom, focus on your thoughts as waves of energy radiating outward from your mind to physical destinations, like your hands and fingers, where they can then generate action that creates material change. Note how before wiping the sleep from your eyes and washing your face, you must first generate thought energy. Next, before powering up your smartphone, think about the waves of energy that make it possible for you to connect with favorite faces and faraway places. Then, as you open your garage and car doors with your remotes, try envisioning the waves of energy that enable you to gain access to your car. This ping-ponging back and forth between energy and apparent matter takes place in your life all day, every day. You're always looking right at energy, you're just perhaps not seeing it. You've been taught to see the appearance of matter.

In his 1915 paper on the theory of relativity that ultimately earned him a Nobel Prize in 1921, Albert Einstein shook the very foundations of Western culture by proving that matter and energy are merely different manifestations of the same thing. Einstein began dismantling the walls of material reality. His genius was poised to shift the global paradigm, yet here we are nearly a century later, and we're still not seeing what we're looking at. In essence, we honored Einstein with a Nobel Prize for opening our eyes to the reality of energy, and then retreated back to our limited Newtonian vision. If Einstein's assertion that energy and matter are one was indeed worthy of the world's Nobel acknowledgment more than ninety years ago, then it would seem high time that our Newtonian blindness should finally be healed.

Nonetheless, classical Newtonian mechanics continues to maintain a loosening grip on the Western world's perception of reality. For many, the ways of matter and energy are still defined in terms of physical laws like gravity. In 1925, however, when Werner Heisenberg advanced his theory of quantum mechanics, all that was radically challenged. Suddenly energy and matter were defined from the energetic level. This shift in perspective shook the very foundations of the Western world's perception of reality.

Look at your hand. Look at the walls around you. Look at the ceiling and the floors above and beneath you. Everything appears to be solid, but now we know that solidity is a phenomenon that only appears to be real. The solid masses that appear before us in the material world are composed of atoms, and the atom is a basic unit of matter that is pure energy. The very building blocks that make up the raw materials of everything before your eyes are merely vibrating fluctuations of energy. In fact, the entire material world you believe you perceive is 99.999 percent pure energy, and only 0.001 percent matter. Regardless of what you and I were taught to believe we're seeing, the fact is, energy is what gives the world the appearance of form.

On July 4, 2012, it was announced that two experiments performed by scientists at the CERN Large Hadron Collider in Geneva, Switzerland, provided 99 percent proof of the discovery of the Higgs boson, or "God particle." Physicists have been searching for this elusive particle since the early 1960s. It is believed to represent the very particle that gives shape and size to all matter and explains mass-energy conversion. This scientific milestone is described by some experts as being as important as the Big Bang theory, because it proves that energy gives the appearance of form to everything material.

Named after physicist Peter Higgs, who first proposed the theory in 1964, the Higgs boson was dubbed the "God particle" by the media following Leon Lederman's book on the topic in 1993. The "God particle" tag may be a bit much for some, but it points to the profound importance of the discovery—the Higgs boson is expected to provide us with a better understanding of how energy gives the appearance of form to all material objects.

THE COLLECTIVE SHIFT

We understand that change is a natural constant. We can observe the changes that take place at the microcosmic level—our weather changes, our community changes, our nation changes, and our world changes, daily, weekly, monthly, and yearly. It's no different at the macrocosmic level—it's just that we can't directly observe it. The galaxy changes, our universe changes, the multiverse changes, and the cosmos changes. The big wheels of change are turning the little wheels. The changes we are currently experiencing are massive in that they are cosmically and universally driven, and they are awakening an expanding consciousness for infinite possibility.

The structure of all known physical laws has always demanded that the universe has only three space dimensions, which include the laws of gravity, radiation, and electromagnetism. Material reality, as we've always known it, has depended on mathematics and physics to advance a three-dimensional theory. The first dimension is defined by the straight line, the second dimension is characterized by the sphere, and the third is defined by the area within a cube.

Our imaginations were previously encoded with this orthodox cognitive downloading, so that most of us were not inclined to stretch our minds beyond the three-dimensional reality. Suddenly everything is changing, as the word *multidimensionalism* has become part of our lexicon. Our collective shift in dimensional reality was inspired by great visionaries.

Noted mathematicians Menaechmus and Apollonius of ancient Greece are believed to have been the first to introduce an analytical geometry that arrived at the coordinates within the infinite space dimension. In the mid-1600s, René Descartes proposed a multidimensional theory based on his understanding of visual-spatial perception. In the 1860s, Friedrich Miescher, Swiss chemist and discoverer of DNA, shocked the scientific community by positing that there were more than three dimensions. Many mathematicians have since proposed similar theories, but it wasn't until the mid-1970s that string theory fully expanded on the idea of multidimensionalism.

Particles appear to have no internal structure, but in the 1970s, string theorists suggested that if we had the technology available for further examination, we'd see that the very particles that make up everything in the universe are not spatially dimensional, or "point like" at all. String advocates claimed that each particle contains a vibrating loop, or string. Strings do things that single points don't. More specifically, they vibrate. String theory posits that the entire universe is made up of vibrating strings that reflect a space reality with up to eleven dimensions. By the 1990s, string theory was extended to include higher-dimensional objects called membranes. This is referred to as M-theory, or membrane theory. M-theory suggests that vibrating strings can evolve into larger vibrating membranes, which can then evolve into entirely new universes. This evolving multiplicity of universes represents an infinite cosmos, with the potential for infinite dimensions.

Our physical universe may have been defined by three-dimensional space, but physics tells us that the larger portion of the universe of "dark matter" is multidimensional. Conventional science has no viable strategy for contending with the concept of multidimensional dark space. Dark space refers to the material region between galaxies. It makes up virtually the entire volume of the universe. It is as undefinable as the inner space within the human mind. There are no boundaries, nor are there any dimensional restrictions that exist in either of these regions. Dark space and inner space represent vastness that transcends 3-D reality.

The multiverse is an infinite domain of pure phenomena, but because we lack the intellectual capacity to observe such limitlessness through standard empirical means, our tendency has always been to assume that it doesn't exist. Quantum mechanics has changed all this by suggesting that any particular phenomenon that can be viewed by an observer is in fact validated by the observer's presence. In short, an observer affects the reality of that which is being observed. What's more, the observer needn't even be human.

In a study recently conducted at the Weizmann Institute of Science in Rehovot, Israel, researchers discovered, with the aid of a chemical electronic electron detector, that observer witnessing was all that was necessary to cause changes in the interference patterns of electron waves. In other words, the device had the same effect on the wave changes as a human observer. Observation by anything causes changes in wave patterns. Both mathematical probability and physics continue to take our collective perception of dimensional reality to new levels.

"Hilbert Space," named after German mathematician David Hilbert in the first decade of the twentieth century, refers to extended methods of calculus and algebra from the three-dimensional space to an infinite number of dimensions. This mathematical approach revealed a theoretical framework with an infinite number of vectors in an abstract space with an infinite number of dimensions. Hilbert space bridges the logic of mathematical probability with the abstract of infinite possibility. A very different level of intellectual thought or consciousness is required to grasp the concept of a multidimensional universe.

American physicist David Bohm advanced a holographic theory of the universe he called the "implicate order," which connects everything with everything else as an unbroken whole, in one undivided movement, with no boundaries. Bohm's theory, intuited from profound insights, begins with his assertion that particles are complete systems with complex internal structures containing detailed information that manifests in quantum wave form. In short, Bohm gave physics a soul. With his implicate order, elementary particles take on animation. These once "robotic" elements suddenly emerge with a "conscious" identity. Bohm identified a unique DNA, spirit, and heartbeat in every particle. Furthermore, he united them, freed them, and perhaps freed us from all restrictive boundaries and dimensions.

A PERSONAL SHIFT

My perception of life has been forever changed. The person I've transformed into over the past thirty years is so radically different, I feel like a Ruth Montgomery "walk-in." I no longer perceive reality in the same way I once did. I was raised to believe that life revolves around living "stuff," and that living "stuff" generates the action that produces energy. I believed the universe to be a domain of forms. There were stars that shone, rivers that flowed, and animals that walked and talked. Mine was a matter-centric reality. Humans represented beings of form that produced energy by thinking, walking, talking, and doing. I was raised to accept that matter preceded—and therefore produced—energy. This all changed as soon as I began to delve into classical Chinese medicine.

Almost immediately after initiating this work, I began to see life from a very different vantage point. Chinese medicine assumes an energy-centric reality and, not unlike Bohm's implicate order, it is based on a universal cosmology of origin, structure, and change. Through the prisms of both Bohm's implicate order and the Chinese medicine hologram, we see past and future, East and West integrated as one. This age-old culture has forever ascribed to the belief that energy represents the unseen source of all things. This ancient quantum wisdom resonated with my innermost instincts and continues to be my greatest source of personal and professional inspiration.

During the course of my early studies, a few basic messages were common threads woven through the fabric of every scintilla of information that I'd encountered. Energy is everywhere. Reality begins with energy. Energy isn't merely the effect, it's the cause. The universe is replete with exactly enough energy. No additional energy is needed, nor can any be added. In fact, if human beings desire more energy, they must learn to cultivate it. They must also attain the wisdom that teaches them to preserve it, rather than waste it.

Now, wherever I turn, everything I hear, smell, touch, and taste I understand to be a manifestation of energy. My perceptions hold true for people as well—I understand that their thoughts, words, actions, and deeds are part of an interwoven mosaic, a panoply of life inextricably tied to a greater matrix of energy. I now also understand that in this universe of energy that gives the illusion of matter, there are unseen, unwritten laws of cause and effect—laws that, once mastered, maximize the balance of our life-force energy.

I was raised to understand life as an unintegrated series of random a priori experiences, events, and circumstances that manifest purely at a material level. Suddenly, I was beginning to see the multiverse from a perspective that views all of life as a holograph of implicate order—integrated, inductive, and energy-based. For the first time in my life I was peering through a lens that revealed all things as energy, flowing into one another, affecting one another, and changing the multiverse.

Let me try to explain this another way. I was guided by constructs that suggested that everything was compartmentalized and separate. I understood there to be four separate seasons: winter, spring, summer, and fall. Then, all at once, I came to understand that the ice masses of winter were also the nurturing flow that would feed the early spring blossoms, and that the warmth of late spring was also the same energy that contributed to the germination of the high grasses of early summer, and so on.

The ancient Chinese perspective reveals an integral model of life where everything is part of a unified energetic holograph. Unlike in the materialistic West, theirs is a vitalistic position deeply rooted in the belief that energy is the true animating "stuff" of life. The two cultures are, quite simply, worlds apart. I found this to be especially true, and most disturbing, in the areas of medicine and healing.

Here in the West, medicine is largely a matter of diagnosing and prescribing. It's all about discovering the disease the patient's symptoms point to, and then finding a pharmaceutical protocol designed to offset those symptoms. In short, it's about treating the symptoms with drugs. The classical Chinese medicine model suggests that there is a causal root for everything, and in order to successfully treat the patient, you must trace the problem back to its root with the intention of eliminating the cause of the imbalance.

For example, the symptoms of pneumonia could be rooted in an overconsumption of phlegmatic foods, such as dairy. If so, dairy foods must be eliminated from the patient's diet in order to free up the blocked lung energy. Where classical Chinese medicine believes that all things are interconnected, they would also be inclined to evaluate the possibility of emotion influencing the root of a physical health problem. For example, the symptoms of pneumonia might also be rooted in an excess of an emotion, such as sadness. By encouraging the patient to express and release the energy of the excess sadness, the lung blockage might then be cleared.

Classical Chinese medicine ascribes to the belief that everything is a manifestation of a great life force called ch'i (energy), and that all forms of ch'i, including emotions and cells, are interconnected. Through 5,000 years of observing the ways of ch'i, the ancient Chinese painstakingly correlated and observed the interconnections of the subtle energy relationships between all things—this wisdom is the great source of inspiration for my personal shift in consciousness. It is what inspired the Whole Health Healing System, and all the healing work I have done to date, as well as all the work I will do in the future. It awakened me to the fact that we are all part of a far greater reality that remains hidden from view and inspired me to dedicate myself to deciphering the natural "ways of a great force," to which we are all inextricably bound.

A GREAT FORCE

Our ancestors had no choice but to attain mastery over the nature that challenged them. From their earliest origins, they were forced to either adapt to unseen energies within and around them or perish. They must have been in awe of the great force that animated life.

All external energetic phenomena—thunder, lightning, rain, snow, fire, the movements of the sun, stars, and planets—stirred their sense of wonder and challenged their ability to cooperate with the laws of nature. The same held true for their relationship with internal energies such as hunger, emotion, intuition, love, and creativity. The demands from all forms of subtle, natural phenomena often tested and threatened their very will to survive. As they evolved, they attained greater wisdom about the ways of energy. This, more than anything, is what enabled them to master the art of survival. The mystical animating force hidden from view both captivated and compelled our ancestors from their earliest beginnings.

In 1868, a hunter from Santander, Spain, accidentally stumbled upon a large cave containing an assemblage of remarkable prehistoric drawings, surmised to be from the Aurignacian civilization, dating back around 700,000 years, to the Middle Paleolithic Era. Many anthropologists believe that these mystical cave murals, with their earthly and surrealistic depictions, represent the earliest evidence of an awareness of life energy.

Our ancient ancestors had an abiding respect and understanding of life energy. Ancient cave wall ruins in India, Egypt, Peru, Europe, and the Yucatán reveal graphic depictions of the human aura. Wherever displayed, the human aura remains a historical constant, an affirmation that energy is indeed at the very core of life.

There are more than 150 words from virtually every language and culture referencing the concept of life energy. According to Hindu tradition, this manifestation of life energy is called Prana. The word *Prana* combines the Sanskrit *Pra* (life) and *Na* (to breathe). Thus, Prana may be translated as "life breath." Ancient Yogic philosophy maintains that Prana radiates as an auric life force from within and around the physical body, reflecting the state of health. The aura is also believed to represent a person's magnetic power of attraction. According to Vedic tradition, this power and magnetism from one's life-force aura may be transmitted to others for the purposes of healing.

The concept of life energy is evident in all ancient cultures. The Egyptians referred to this energy as *Ka*, the Tibetans called it *La*; the ancient Hebrews used the term *Ruah*. Ancient American Indian tribes also developed a language to facilitate the concept of life energy. The Lakota Sioux of the western plains referred to life energy as *Woniya Wakan*, or "Holy Air." The Cree people of the woodlands and plains of the United States and Canada called it *Oenikika*, or "Breath of Life."

Native South American tribes were no different from their Native North American brothers. They too understood and revered the concept of life energy. The Mayans called it *Ik*, which translates as "Breath of Life," while the Aztecs spoke of *Tona*, "Vital Heat."

The Polynesians referred to the great energy as Manna. In Hawaii, indigenous healers still embrace the concept that Manna gives life. It has been a long-held, sacred tradition of Hawaiians to train their shamans and medicine men (kahunas) to cultivate and transmit the Manna life energy to those most in need of healing. In accordance with ancient kahuna belief, the subconscious mind attempts to channel life force to the "will" for purposes of ego gratification, whereas the higher mind seeks to direct the force for the higher good of spiritual transformation and healing. This is similar to the ancient teachings of Chinese *Fang-Chung-Shu* (bedroom arts) and Hindu Kundalini Yoga that a libidinal life energy—Shakti in Hindu philosophy—lies dormant in the sexual organs. This powerful sexual energy can be directed upward to fuel the higher centers of awareness through the practice of Kundalini Yoga. Once mastered, the discipline ascends one's life force beyond the ego, to the spirit.

The Kung San of the African Kalahari Desert refer to life energy as *Num*. They believe that Num is stored both in the lower abdomen and at the base of the spine, and that the best way to circulate the life-giving Num to the body, mind, and spirit is to make it "boil," by way of ceremonial dance. Once "boiled" and circulated, Num is believed to imbue the body with vibrant health, the mind with emotional balance, and the spirit with consummate wisdom.

As a lifelong student of natural healing, I was always drawn to the idea of tracing the origins of disease back as far as they could go. Therefore it was a natural transition for me to accept the theory that life begins at the subtlest energetic level. When I initiated my work some years later, I began an immediate search for some kind of model "whole-istic" system of medicine that was energy-based. Though I discovered that there were many, there was one in particular that attracted my attention.

I learned that when Chinese medicine refers to "ch'i," it is referring simply to the agent that gives life to all living things, and is perhaps the most fundamentally important word in the Chinese language. The Chinese believe that ch'i animates and permeates the universe and gives breath to life. In terms of human health, ch'i is the life energy that enables blood to circulate, glands to secrete, and metabolism to function. The only reason the human heart beats is that ch'i dwells within the body. Once devoid of ch'i, the body is but an empty shell. This is central to the concept of Chinese energy healing—we can either choose to cultivate an abundance of life energy or we can carelessly allow our life energy to slip away.

VIBRATION: THE DANCE OF
THE GREAT FORCE

An abundance of life energy makes for a healthy living being. Healthy living beings reflect vitality. Vitality is represented by movement. When we speak in energy terms we must think of vitality and movement as possessing vibration. The difference between life and death is vibration. The difference between levels of vitality is vibration.

Everything is energy, and energy is always moving. The fundamental movement of energy is called vibration. Vibration is an oscillatory response that reflects greater and lesser degrees of energy in action. At the subatomic level, beyond the illusion of matter, nothing rests. Particles, atoms, molecules, and cells continuously vibrate at an infinite variety of ever-changing frequencies. Therefore, everything appearing to be standing still is in fact constantly vibrating. You and I are vibrating right now!

The concept of vibration has special significance in virtually every aspect of life, especially health and healing. For most of us, the notion of health and medicine remains purely a material proposition. Medical orthodoxy may employ energy-based technologies like magnetic resonance imaging and ultrasound, but when it comes to translating the results, it's all mechanical. The patient is seen as a mass of material biology, and the solution is either a surgeon's blade or a pill. So what about energy and vibration? Beyond MRIs and ultrasound machines, can we actually come to better understand energy vibration in ways that enable us to kill viruses, heal disease, and improve our health?

In the early twentieth century, bioelectric researcher Georges Lakhovsky was among the first to theorize that all cells vibrate, exhibiting all the properties required of an oscillator: inductance, capacitance, and resistance. Lakhovsky postulated that all living cells were both transmitters and receivers of high-frequency oscillations. He further theorized that all living cells vibrate at different frequencies and surmised that viruses oscillate at different frequencies than healthy human cells. When the virus attacks the healthy cell, the cell can't defend itself from the more powerful viral vibration. If the amplitude, or energy potential, of the healthy cell becomes compromised, and that of the virus becomes stronger, more severe illness will result. By returning a specific cell to its homeostasis frequency, Lakhovsky thought that one could both antagonize the frequency of disease and restore the healthy cell to balance.

Following the work of Lakhovsky, American inventor Dr. Royal Raymond Rife spent three decades studying specific vibrational "kill" frequencies of hundreds of microorganisms. As far back as 1920, Rife theorized that disease-causing microorganisms vibrated at specific oscillation rates, and that if these were better understood, they might be safely eliminated by an opposing rate of vibration.

With his expertise in optics, Rife developed microscopes with resolutions up to 17,000 times in diameter compared to the standard 2,500. With the aid of his high-powered microscopes, Rife methodically observed and cataloged the results, as he exposed pathogenic microorganisms to coordinated resonance from electronic frequencies. During his thirty years of vibrational research, Rife established what he called the Mortal Oscillatory Rate (MOR) for hundreds of disease-causing pathogens.

In his work, Rife confirmed thousands of living vibrational frequencies. He determined that the average frequency of a healthy human body was between 62 and 72 Hz and that when the frequency drops below this average, it signifies a compromised immune system. He established that the human brain frequency ranges between 4 and 30 Hz, and the human heart between 67 and 70 MHz. Rife further discovered that colds and flu begin at 57–60 MHz, *Candida* fungal overgrowth at 55 MHz, Epstein-Barr virus at 52 MHz, cancer at 42 MHz, and death at 25 MHz. Rife also noted that fresh organic foods vibrated at an average of 20–30 Hz, higher than processed and/or dried foods, and that essential oils can register as high as 320 Hz. He claimed that therapeutic-grade essential oils have the highest frequency of any natural substance known to man.

Rife meticulously mapped out a living mosaic of energy vibration, but he was simply too far ahead of his time to be appreciated for his contribution. By determining the vibration rate of cancer cells and further claiming that he'd successfully killed cancer cells, both his unfortunate timing and his cancer cure claims made him a political enemy of the healing establishment. For decades, the orthodoxy castigated and ridiculed Rife as a charlatan. As is often the case, the more time goes by, the more a man's genius is understood enough to be appreciated. Not surprisingly, the scientific community managed to come full circle, right back to where Rife's work left off.

On January 18, 1941, a University of Pennsylvania study appeared in the *Journal of General Physiology* that bore a striking resemblance to the research that Rife had done a decade earlier. This particular study, entitled "The Effect of Sonic Vibrations on Phage, Phage Precursor, and the Bacterial Substrate," studied the effects of oscillated sonic and ultrasonic vibrations on vaccinia viruses and *Staphylococcus* bacterial substrates. The intention was to rupture and inactivate viral and bacterial cells with quartz crystal–generated vibrations set at frequencies between 8,900 and 9,300 cycles per second. The study did note vibrational disruption and deactivation of pathogens.

More recently, in September 2009, researchers at MIT measured the varied frequencies at which healthy human red blood cells and infectious malaria cells vibrate. This research supported Rife's contention that cells have electrochemical as well as biological activity within, producing nanoscale vibrational frequencies. This research represents a kind of "Rife-like" game changer. In a world where mutated and engineered germs are about to make current material medicines outdated and ineffective, vibrational medicine may be the medicine of a future that has already arrived.

In 2012, researchers at Arizona State University mathematically determined the frequencies at which viruses could be energetically shaken to death. Viruses have a capsid shield that insulates and protects them. These researchers have discovered that by aggressively vibrating a virus, they can break down its protective shield and the virus can be easily killed.

Researchers at the University of California at Los Angeles recently discovered that even baker's yeast cells vibrate—at a rate of 1,000 times per second. The researchers noted that their motions were too fast to be captured on video but once converted to sound waves they were found to generate what scientists referred to as a high-pitched scream recorded at two octaves above true middle C.

This research presents us with an entirely different way of viewing life, disease, and medicine. Everything is energy, energy vibrates, and all energy vibrates at its own unique frequency. We in the West are at last poised to master this reality that transcends matter. Unlike disease, humans have the power to willfully transmit vibration—vibration that antagonizes disease.

THOUGHT VIBRATION: THE DANCING MIND

Everything vibrates. Every particle, atom, molecule, and cell within us vibrates. The vibrational centers of our being are our mind and brain. The brain is made up of around 100 billion neurons with trillions of synaptic connections. Each signal is capable of up to 1,000 signals per second, producing an average of 300–3,000 thoughts per minute. Neurons fire at approximately 250 miles per hour as they transmit thought impulses. When the synaptic charge reaches its receptor, it triggers cascades of neurochemicals. Once this synaptic response is completed, physical causality manifests in the form of thought. Beyond this physical, quantifiable reality, things get small, very small. Thoughts are smaller than 100 nanometers (one billionth of a meter) long. This characterizes thought as occurring at the quantum level. Thoughts have been described by quantum theorists as microbursts that generate electromagnetic fields of energy that vibrate to cognizance, and pass like collapsing waves. Beyond these physical and quantum levels, the causal nature of thought is indeterminable. Beyond the causal curtain, there is a higher power that is the source of vibration.

Scientists can now read a person's thoughts with the aid of an MRI (magnetic resonance imaging) machine. They've found that when a subject views common images his brain produces identifiable vibrational patterns. Moreover, vibrations triggered from deep emotional states and higher creative ideas have their own distinctive vibrational identity. Beyond the realm of the physical and the quantum causality, higher thought—such as compassion and love—produces a much higher vibration, capable of producing "peak experiences," or transpersonal states.

In February 2012, fifteen-year-old Austin Smith and his seventy-four-year-old grandfather, Ernest Monhollen, were repairing Austin's Buick when the car suddenly slipped off of the cinder blocks and landed squarely on top of Ernest. Austin swiftly lifted the car with his bare hands and moved it off his grandfather, saving his life. Afterward, Austin credited his deep, abiding love for his "Papa Ernie" as the motivation for his heroic deed. The boy's actions defied logic at every level. His emotions clearly opened the door to a "peak experience." This experience and many others like it prove that higher thoughts vibrate energy from a place within us that is unrestricted by limitation.

Until very recently, the human energy–based anatomy generated seven different vibrational frequencies. Due to recent cosmic astrological shifts, there are now six additional higher frequencies.

We generate conscious energies from as low as survival to as high as divine.

Some time ago, I saw a young woman diagnosed with multiple sclerosis (MS) who gave a testimonial on a YouTube documentary of mine called *Choosing to Live*. When we first met, I explained to her that her condition was largely the result of a genetic expression triggered in part by stress. I pointed out that MS, being a neurode-generative (nerve-degenerating) disease, has been proven to advance more aggressively when coupled with acute stress. I then explained that acute stress typically results in powerful negative engrams (trapped memory patterns) in the unconscious mind that continue to transmit neurodegenerative brain signals. This constant flow of stress signals overdrives the nerve pathways, further eroding the insulating myelin sheath. Simply translated, the emotional energy from long-term stress wears out your physical/material body. As I so often do, I gave her some powerful mind-reformatting exercises for homework. Neuroplasticity research continues to prove that positive mind-reformatting exercises rehearsed with regularity can, over time, reformat and help regenerate nerve pathways. The woman has been both medication- and MS-symptom free for more than twenty years now. She attributes her success to her positive mind-reformatting work.

Most of the patients I see these days are very different from those I have seen over the years. The level of consciousness and spiritual sophistication of today's patient far exceeds that of a patient from a decade ago. Today's patients are much more in touch with their inner knowing. They also have a greater desire to be "inner known."

I recently visited with a patient who suffers from anaphylactic shock episodes that routinely send her off to the emergency room. She told me that while many medicines were prescribed for her condition, none proved to be of safe, functional value. She shared an interesting story with me. She told me that the root of her problem is that she is far too emotionally sensitive and empathic to the pain of others and that recently, while consoling a friend in great pain, she took on the stress of her friend to such a degree that she actually brought on an anaphylactic episode in herself. She then explained that she had effectively overcome her condition by reformatting her mind through positive thought exercises. She told me that sixteen weeks of positive mental imagery, for ten minutes per day, was enough to help her reduce her episodes by 90 percent. Consciousness and mind power did what medicine simply could not do.

Consciousness is the greatest power in the universe (with due respect, perhaps, to supermassive black holes and gamma-ray bursts). Consciousness has the power to generate love, compassion, intelligence, and self-reflection. Moreover, consciousness with *intention* produces an energy field of pure potential and infinite possibility— a higher-thermodynamic, free energy, which can generate enough power to produce virtually any effect, even miracle healing.

In his book *Reinventing Medicine*, Larry Dossey writes, "Approximately 150 studies support the ability of thoughts, wishes, and prayers to affect distant biological systems. These experiments not only involve humans but human tissue that has been removed from the body, as well as animals, plants, and microorganisms."

We all have the power to heal with our thoughts. Healing thought vibrations are things, things that know not the restrictions of time and space.

THOUGHTS DANCING THROUGH
INFINITE SPACE

Thoughts are pulsed electrical charges within the bioelectrical circuitry of the brain. In accordance with quantum entanglement, where energies act upon one another coactively, all pulsed electrical charges generate information. Therefore, thought-based information is a form of matter that's continually shared at billions of times the speed of light in the quantum vacuum of zero point. A simpler way of looking at this fact is that every thought everyone has ever had is continually being shared with the entire universe. The universe is like a large brain that receives and processes the total sum of all information. Our thoughts identify us as microuniverses that share our information with the macrouniverse. When it comes to our thoughts, we are all part of a universal shared library plan.

There are two ways for us to share our thoughts, unconsciously and consciously. Regardless of whether or not we intend to share our thoughts, they are information that is transmitted and shared via quantum entanglement. We may, however, consciously make our thoughts intentional, and direct them to specific sources.

All atoms produce electromagnetic fields. Thoughts are comprised of atoms. Thought generates low frequencies that emit vibrating waves. The human brain generally produces frequencies in the range of 4–30 Hz, which is a lower exponent of the extremely low radio frequency or ELF range (3–30 KHz) once used to communicate with submarines. We are all designed by nature to communicate via thought, and not just at the sensory level, but at the supersensory energetic level.

Unconscious thought-wave vibrations are omnidirectional—they're transmitted in all directions. Conscious intentions, however, generate a far more powerful wave vibration and are unidirectional—they're transmitted in only one direction.

Over the past thirty years, I have transmitted a tremendous amount of distance healing to a number of subjects with great effectiveness. Even as the world insisted on debating the matter, I chose to further develop my distance healing skills. Today I continue to successfully perform nonlocal healing on patients from all around the world. Recently I transmitted a form of distance healing called Wenchiech'u (an ancient Chinese healing discipline) to two patients with severe cases of sciatica. I requested that they forward me e-mails regarding their condition within a week. They both informed me that their pain had completely abated overnight.

I shall never forget the very first patient I ever worked with "nonlocally." A woman from Ireland, whose sister I'd worked with for years, asked if I'd be willing to do some distance healing work with her. She was experiencing severe migraine headaches at the time, and was feeling desperate. She'd tried everything imaginable, to no avail. I remember feeling quite intimidated by her request. My intellectual self was fine with the idea, as I clearly understood the quantum mechanics of it all, but actually doing it would be a true test to my belief. I agreed not to charge her any fee, and we proceeded.

First, she gave me a brief history of her health and reported that she was suffering from a severe migraine as we spoke. She went on to explain that as a young child, she was emotionally abused at home, as well as routinely tormented by the children she often played with. This stayed with me throughout our conversation. We spoke for no more than twenty minutes before I began sending her a healing intention. Initially I had great trouble concentrating, but I eventually settled in. The critical factor that enabled me to inten- sify my focus was the compassion I felt from hearing of her child- hood abuse. It created a truly intense power of compassionate intention within me. Just before hanging up the phone she reported that her headache had completely cleared. I have since learned that for me, compassion makes a profound difference when it comes to effective distance healing. We worked together for years and I am happy to report that she remained headache free throughout our time together.

In *Reinventing Medicine*, Larry Dossey refers to three eras in medicine—Era I is described as material, mechanical, or physical medicine like surgery or prescription; Era II refers to local mind/ body medicine, like hypnosis, biofeedback, positive thinking, and psychoneuroimmunology; and Era III medicine is where mind is a key factor, but at long distances, such as intercessory prayer. Era III is best characterized as any intervention that includes a consciousness bridge between people at any distance. Era III medicine implies that we have the power to heal with our nonlocal mind. Nonlocal mind is just what it sounds like. The mind isn't the brain. The brain is a biological organ stuck in place right between the ears. The mind isn't located in any one place, nor does it operate with local restriction. The mind is a potential transmitter of distance healing intentions.

THE GREATEST FORCE: AN INFINITE MIND

As I interface with my patients every day, the subtle undercurrents of their energies are palpable to me. There is so much diverse life force vibrating in each and every one of them. I can feel the bio-electricity of their bodies, minds, hearts, and spirits. I can sense their willingness and their resistance. I can feel the rising currents from deep within their thoughts and shifting moods. I sense their responsiveness to the sea of life energy that surrounds them. They may react with great sensitivity to the power of a simple word in conversation or to a stream of sunlight as it glistens in the room. The sound vibrations emanating from the background music in the room may unexpectedly prompt an old, forgotten memory from the depths of their unconscious mind. They are so much more than mere physical entities. Each and every one is a unique universe of ever-changing infinite energy.

What many of my patients suffer from is a separation from their own energetic being. Everywhere they go and in everything they do, they are objectified into believing that they are mere material bodies. I can't help but notice how responsive most of them are while communicating at a deeper, energetic level. There is so much more to them than the depreciated images they've been cognitively indoctrinated with.

The daily depictions of life that so falsely define their worth are partially responsible for the anomie and dis-ease that so many of them suffer from. Life itself is routinely portrayed as having little or no worth. Ours has degenerated into a "drive-by" society. By the time a child finishes elementary school, he or she has observed 8,000 murders on television. The constant objectification, abuse, and sterilized extinguishing of life has become entertainment and sport. We have become experts at making our minds and our thoughts dis-eased, but we have also begun to turn the corner. The changes that have begun to take place in the world's collective consciousness clearly deliver a profoundly different message about who we truly are and what we're really capable of.

The overwhelmingly positive results from my healing work with patients have made it very clear to me that people are beginning to transform their minds and thoughts. They are beginning to discover the unlimited energy potentials of their infinite minds.

On July 27, 2008, in an interview that is part of *The Life Energy of Consciousness* video documentary, William Tiller, professor emeritus of material sciences and engineering at Stanford, said, "The vacuum within a single hydrogen atom has 30 trillion times more energy than there is in all of the mass of all of the stars and all the planets up to 20 billion light-years. If consciousness were to allow you to control a small fraction of that energy, then creating a big bang would be no problem." This suggests that the currency for energy is consciousness, and that there is no limit to what is available!

Imagine a new reality where thoughts alone have the potential to be powerful agents of material change. Imagine a reality where, by merely massing enough conscious intention, one could generate enough higher-thermodynamic free energy in a vacuum to heal a friend of a disease a thousand miles away. Regardless of what we continue to believe, we're beginning to discover that the limitations of material reality are vanishing right before our very eyes. Our former reality baselines are giving way to new vistas without boundaries.

Noted mind/body medicine pioneer Dr. Herbert Benson once headed up a series of amazing research projects sponsored by the Harvard Medical School. One study in particular was aimed at documenting the mind power of Tibetan monks in the Himalayas, where for many thousands of years there have been reports of an extraordinary mind/body ceremony.

Dr. Benson and his research crew set out to study one particular group of Tibetan Buddhists who practiced a meditation ceremony called Tum-Mo Yoga, which is said to help them generate such concentrated thought power that they can actually elevate their skin energy for the express purpose of drying their robes in the frigid temperatures of their mountaintop monastery. With an indoor temperature of only forty degrees, each monk stripped off his clothing, except for a small loincloth. The monks assumed a full lotus position, wrapped in forty-nine-degree, sopping-wet garments as they began to practice their mind-altering yoga. Benson's crew watched in amazement as the monks put on their cold, wet robes and calmly sat without flinching. Within three to five minutes, the camera lenses of Benson's film crew began to fog up. The scientists reported that their lenses had to constantly be wiped dry. In thirty minutes, the monks and their once-cold, wet robes were both perfectly warm and dry. Benson's crew successfully filmed and documented the entire remarkable proceeding.

Energy manifests as two conceptual realities—physical reality at the atomic, molecular level and consciousness reality at the vacuum level. The physical reality that has presided over life to date is beginning to give way to consciousness reality. The collective awareness of our world is swiftly transiting through a dramatic shift in awareness. Transformational consciousness is leading many to deeper levels of discovery. It's no longer just about the particles, atoms, molecules, cells, and material bodies. It's becoming more about the unlimited energy potential in the space between them. Tiller reminds us that it's the higher-thermodynamic free energy states of thought and intention that govern material reality, and ultimately drive all processes, from our physical bodies to all that surrounds them.

THE GREAT FORCE IS ALWAYS WITH US

Twenty years ago I counseled a woman who was diagnosed with end-stage breast cancer. I will refer to her as Rita. I will never forget the day Rita first walked into my office. She had a distant look in her eye. Her head was tilted off to the side as if she didn't want to make direct eye contact. She was smiling and seemed as though she was not fully connected with the gravity of her situation. I asked her if she was all right. All she continued to say was, "I'm not going to go anywhere." I was convinced that the stress of her ordeal was weighing heavily on her mental equilibrium. Nonetheless, she continued to remind me that she wasn't going to go anywhere. A week later she arrived at my office unexpectedly, with a camera. I reminded her that she didn't have a scheduled appointment. She said that she came only to take a quick snapshot of me. I obliged and she said she'd be back in a week.

Sure enough, she reappeared a week later with a collage that included a picture of myself, her nurse-practitioner neighbor, her health food store proprietor, and her acupuncturist, among others. Rita had put together a team photo of all her caregivers. She wanted each of us to have a copy so we could all be synced into an energy loop together. Suddenly I began to realize that Rita wasn't crazy at all. Quite the contrary—Rita was building an energetic ring of fire around herself from which to draw strength. Soon thereafter, Rita was declared cancer free. I've received a thank-you card from her every year during the holiday season for more than twenty years now. Rita taught me a very valuable lesson: It's not about cells and pills. When you get right down to it, life and healing are about energy.

Energy has become the cornerstone of my life and health care practice. Everything I do is based on energy. I train my interns in this same spirit. I begin by reformatting their thinking. Understanding that they have been inculcated to accept the limitations of a material reality, I teach them to shift their thinking to a more extrasensory level of perception. I begin by telling them that a practitioner of Whole Health Healing must never wait until physically interfacing with the patient to engage their intake and evaluation. I demand that they tune into their patients upon first greeting them. I encourage them to look into their eyes in search of energy, and to really tap into the life force of the hand they're shaking. I know they are becoming accomplished when they can tune into their patients as they approach the building from the parking lot. The practitioners of Whole Health must live life at a very different level—they must come to think of themselves as receptors and transmitters of energy that have the capability of tuning in at much deeper levels than they are accustomed to.

Current systems of natural health care embrace the concept of disease prevention—everything manifests from the subtle to the dense. When a stone is cast into the water, waves ripple from the inside out. In this same spirit, disease manifests from the subtlest energies of mind and spirit to denser symptoms of the physical body. Before disease becomes physical, it must take root as dis-ease at the subtle energetic level. I can't tell you how many thousands of times I have seen asthma that was rooted in grief from the loss of a loved one. I continue to see liver diseases born from lifelong anger, kidney diseases rooted in decades of fear, and pancreatic conditions caused by years of anxiety. If we are ever to master the art of preventive health care, we must first commit to becoming more attuned to the subtle energies that speak of dis-ease in the language of the body. In order to do this we must first come to master the art of living life at the energetic level. Accomplished practitioners of Whole Health healing must transform themselves back into the energetically conscious beings they were designed to be, so that they can be who they are, wherever they are, not merely while at work.

INNER KNOWING:
MASTERY OF THE GREAT FORCE

We don't have to be mathematicians or physicists to know that energy brings form to all material objects. We can best master energy by simply observing life around us from a place deep within us. For example, we might think of ourselves as material objects that can be altered by form-changing energies, such as french fries. If we over-consume french fries, the dense caloric energy will store as fat, which will then expand our waistline and change our physical form. The point here is that energy merely represents a different way of looking at life and, though complex, it can be viewed much more simply from the place of our innermost instincts. Our place of "inner knowing" is the ideal place for observing and demystifying energy.

By his own admission, Einstein possessed only average mathematical skills. He said that many of his most-lauded conclusions were rarely the result of any long calculations, claiming that his memory was too deficient and that any truly accomplished calculation requires an exceptional memory. He claimed that he arrived at most results through his intuitive instinct, a sense of inner knowing as to what the results simply "should be."

Just observe the mutable dynamism of energy within and around you. When you feel emotion, observe the changing energy. When you drink water to quench your thirst, observe the changing energy. When you see the sun shifting the shadows in the room, observe the changing energy. When you embrace someone you love, observe the changing energy.

Our matter-based reality programming has resulted in what I like to call a state of "outer believing." Every culture instills a sense of outer believing in its people for the perceived benefit of the greater good. It's certainly been the case for us. After all, we are a material-based, free-enterprise society that depends on material goods and services for our very survival. The economic powers that be have managed to further reinforce our collective outer believing with the help of the Madison Avenue power machine. More than ever, material marketing and advertising reinforce our outer belief in a matter-based reality, in spite of the transformational discoveries of physics.

To most, physics brings an awkward argument that goes against everything they've been taught to believe in. As enlightening as it has been, it's merely too unapproachable ever to have been a catalyst for cultural change. If we as a culture are ever to benefit from the possibilities of an energy-based reality, such an advantage will have to come from our own simple observations and inner knowing.

The more you observe energy, the more you begin to realize that even though it may escape your five senses, it always exerts powerful effects on them. Energy may be a phenomenon studied by the world's greatest minds, but energy also reflects actionable changes that can be routinely observed by us all. All we have to do is practice seeing it.

Energy is so much more than the words on the pages of a physics textbook. Energy is constantly manifesting within, around, and through our lives, forever altering our form and movement. Observe energy as it infinitely adds and subtracts from your reality. Allow it to inspire an opening of the window to your inner knowing. It's all about seeing what you're looking at. To some, being hit on the head by an apple falling from a tree is much ado about nothing. But to Isaac Newton, it was good enough for a paradigm shift that would eternally change the modern world.

CHAPTER 2

ENERGETIC INDIVIDUALITY

CONSTITUTIONS

A code is a specialized language that translates specific, unique information. One of the greatest examples of this is our genetic code, the language that defines and disseminates the unique information contained within our DNA. Similarly, Whole Health asserts that we each possess our own personal energy codes that can be broken down into a language, which represents all the unique information that makes us who and what we truly are. Whole Health refers to these exclusive energy codes as our constitution.

I recently enjoyed an interesting conversation with a pediatric nurse regarding human constitutions. We chatted for a few moments about my writing this chapter. Our discussion immediately moved into the area of human variation. As we spoke, we drifted off a bit onto the topic of reincarnation. I questioned whether he believed in it, and if so whether he felt it might play a role in the uniqueness of our constitutions. He said that after more than a decade of attending to the birth of "preemies"—premature babies—he was inclined to believe that every single one had come into this world with a fully developed and unique inner core. He said that to his way of thinking, when it comes to the question of nature versus nurture, it was all about nature. He went on to further emphasize how, when you look into their eyes, each preemie reveals a separate, secret universe. As we parted, I reflected on the paradox of energy—how unique yet similar everything is.

I've often thought about the sense of oneness that orbiting astronauts must feel as they gaze down upon Mother Earth from miles up in space. From their lofty macrocosmic perspective, the galaxy appears as a holograph. Observing life at a quantum level, however, provides a glimpse of a world of tiny particles telling a completely different story about the profound uniqueness of all things that are as one. The way of energy is undivided yet sui generis.

We are all as unique as the droplets that make up the same sea of energy. Separation is an illusion, yet the multiverse's varied manifestations remain but a reflection of its unanimity and flux. Even though we are constituents of the same sea, your energy is different from mine. Our energy is different today than it was yesterday, and it will continue to change throughout the course of any given moment, day, week, month, and year. Our subtle flow of constant changes is due to the myriad of mutable energetic influences within and around us, influences such as our thoughts, the food we eat, the people we encounter, the things we do, and the ever-fluctuating conditions we face.

Identical twins may possess the same DNA, and may physically appear to be exactly the same. But at the energetic level, their constitutions are worlds different. Just ask the people who know and love them. Their tastes in food, music, and fashion are likely to be very different. Their moods, emotions, thoughts, and behaviors are also likely to be very different. People are often puzzled when I muscle-test them for food allergies and find they are allergic to lemon but not lime, or to Savoy cabbage but not Chinese cabbage. Because we are accustomed to observing the vicissitudes of life from a purely material, and not an energetic, perspective, we tend to overlook the dynamic, phenomenological variability within and around us. The multiverse may be one, but everything contained within is representative of a separate, complete multiverse.

I recently watched a daytime health-talk show, and as usual the "experts" were hyping a superdetox formula that was touted as being good for everyone. It truly amazes me how stuck we are on the "one size fits all" mentality. It's likely due to the never-ending marketing pipeline that finds its way directly from the research lab to the media outlets and straight to you. While this mind-shaping hype machine may generate an endless stream of revenue, it continually spews obsolete misinformation. No *one* nutritional supplement, drug, or food can be good for everyone. When we're dealing with living energy, every living thing has its own separate constitution.

We are all unique and should never allow ourselves to be cattle-prodded into the corral of "one size fits all" living. We're all forced to contend with our constitution every day; we're simply not aware of it. Some of us look good in yellow while others look good in red. Some of us are drawn to sweet, doughy foods while others prefer salty foods with a crunch. We're each one of a kind, and we all express individual tendencies that reveal our constitution. Whole Health teaches that the first step to true wholeness is to appreciate the subtle energetic differences between all forms.

Over the years I have witnessed many examples of constitutional differences among my patients. For example, a woman once told me that she could only correct her hyperacidity with foods like red meat. Red meat is an acidic food, but for some it may actually help absorb excess hydrochloric acid. I recall another woman who insisted that whenever she consumes peppermint tea with any regularity, she tends to lose weight. Then there was a man who once claimed that he could only regulate his pH (acid/alkaline balance) by consuming a baked potato once a day. We are all microuniverses unto ourselves, together making up a vast macromultiverse. Everywhere you look there are reminders of the multiplicity of constitutions. Recently, the topic of cellular memory theory has provided some interesting perspective regarding the uniqueness of our codes.

As far back as the early 1970s, many heart transplant recipients were noted as having undergone dramatic personality changes that eerily reflected the personality of the donors. Changes in opinion, craving, taste, attitude, and even vocabulary have all been consistently noted in many organ transplant recipients. In his book *The Heart's Code*, neuropsychologist Paul Pearsall tells the story of a three-year-old Arab girl who received the heart of an eight-year-old Jewish boy. One day the girl mysteriously began asking for a type of rare Jewish candy that neither she nor her family had ever heard of, a candy that had been a favorite of the little boy who was her donor. But the concept of our energetic uniqueness isn't just logical, nor is it complicated. We need only turn to common, day-to-day life scenarios to see our personal energy codes revealed.

Imagine going to a party with a good number of invitees. Over the course of the next several hours you will have the opportunity to meet and chat with many of them. The next morning, as you reflect back on your various party encounters, you will likely recall a blend of great, good, fair, poor, and not so great connections. No one personality jibes with all others. Energy must match in order for there to be compatibility. At the subtle energetic level, life is a game of pitch and catch. Some connections spark instantly, some spark a little, and some don't spark at all. And so it is also true when it comes to the mixing and matching energies between people, jobs, music, movies, food, vitamins, and medicine. It's all about constitutions.

Whole Health is a healing system that focuses on the profound differentiation of energy and the exchange of energetic influences from one moment to the next. The thing that truly distinguishes this from other healing systems is that it provides the practitioner with tools to decode and master the art of understanding the energetic constitution.

Our energy codes contain and reflect our own, unique information. At an energy level we all have different quirks, needs, preferences, and tendencies—and we also possess distinctly different spirits, psychologies, and physiologies. Science is beginning to find constitutionality showing up in the most unexpected places.

In June 2012, the Human Microbiome Project published its long-awaited findings, announcing the discovery that we each have our own personal bacterial codes. As it turns out, we all have varying amounts of good and bad bacteria, with a variety of different strains. Moreover, none of our good and bad bacterial populations exhibit the same behaviors. The researchers found that healthy people have "bad" bacteria floating around inside their intestines that live in perfect harmony with their "good" bacteria. They surmised that each bacterial immune system deciphers its own unique way of figuring out how to acclimate itself to the host body. This remarkable research suggests that each of us produces an immunological adaptation reflective of our personal code.

Our constitution codes represent all our most vital information, and in order for us to maximize our balance and wellness, it's essential that we understand the inner workings of our codes. Whole Health asserts that constitution is a vital missing ingredient in our current health care approach. Wellness and disease prevention have become main focuses of medicine, yet we've made no real effort to properly educate patients about their constitutional self. The average patient knows little about good nutrition and even less about their own body, mind, and spirit. When it comes to fixing our broken health care system, patient education in constitution coding might be a good place to start.

In order for each of us to become more willing participants in our own disease prevention, we must become more attuned to our specific individual needs. Without a greater understanding of constitution, there can be no disease prevention. Before we can truly become well as a nation, we must first recover from our chronic "one size fits all" hangover.

I continue to hear patients complain that when they leave my office following food allergy testing, they return to their families, friends, and work associates, only to be grilled by them with unending questions about not being able to eat certain foods—"But I thought dairy had calcium," and "What's wrong with whole wheat?" These questions only reflect a culture that has been programmed to view life solely from a homogenous perspective. To most, energy coding may not seem like such an important issue, but it represents a shift in consciousness that will enable us to take a quantum leap far beyond the imbalanced state of our present health care and lifestyle models.

I have counseled thousands of people whose health conditions were previously either misdiagnosed or simply missed altogether, because the nuances of their personal energy codes were not deciphered. I once worked with a young boy who was dealing with life-threatening anaphylactic peanut allergies. When a few of his teammates on the soccer field decided it wouldn't be a big deal to give him a cookie with a few peanuts in it, they soon discovered that they were very wrong. The boy was rushed to the emergency room, but passed away a short time later.

His was an immunoglobulin E allergy (IgE). This type of food allergy is rare and represents only 1.5 percent of all food allergy reactions, but, as the anecdote illustrates, it is potentially fatal. Meanwhile, some experts estimate that as many as 80–90 million Americans suffer from less-threatening immunoglobulin G (IgG) food allergies. IgG allergies are the causal root of gas, bloating, constipation, and headaches, among many other ailments, but what's more significant is that they are often major contributing factors to a variety of more serious conditions. The most important point of all this is that some 80 percent of those with IgG allergies remain undiagnosed. The reason why we are failing to reach beyond these health limitations is our lack of energy awareness, and the absence of personal coding.

The recent defeat of Proposition 37 in the state of California represents a potential violation of personal coding. This failed referendum establishes a chilling precedent destined to spawn great regret in the not-too-distant future.

Currently, 85 percent of the corn and 91 percent of the soybeans grown in America are genetically modified. About 70 percent of food products on grocery store shelves contain at least one genetically modified ingredient. In many cases, these foods are being bioengineered to include ingredients from other foods. For example, manufacturers have experimented with splicing a gene from deepwater fish into strawberries. Many thousands of years of survival specialization has allowed deepwater fish to develop a protective gene that keeps them from freezing to death. Bioengineering researchers are now looking to splice the fish's antifreezing gene into strawberries to prevent spoilage. Sounds all well and good, but what about those strawberry consumers who are allergic to fish?

California's Proposition 37 would have required labeling for all genetically modified foods. In my opinion, this would have given consumers and emergency room doctors the advantage of vital information in the event of a potentially life-threatening anaphylactic allergic reaction.

Two weeks prior to the vote, polls revealed that 82 percent of Californians were in favor of labeling. But Monsanto and Pepsi were convinced that such labeling would be a public relations nightmare that would cost them millions of dollars in net losses. Thus, following a two-week, multimillion-dollar media blitz by the two industry giants that threatened to pass on astronomical costs to the consumer, the proposition went down in flames. This dark episode has made it perfectly clear that our health care is in our own hands.

THE POWER OF CONSTITUTION CODING

According to the U.S. Department of Health and Human Services, there are 770,000 adverse drug reaction injuries and/or deaths each year, tallying up a cost of over $5.6 million per hospital. In addition, there are millions of adverse reactions to foods and food additives annually in America. Imagine what it might be like if we had a better grasp of the concept of constitution coding. A greater appreciation for the uniqueness of constitution codes would surely save untold lives and dollars. Establishing coding guidelines and educating the general public and health care establishment on the topic of constitutional tendencies would undoubtedly improve the sorry state of our present health care system.

There are but two ways to practice medicine—prevention and intervention. The present medical mantra of "early intervention" should be superseded by a mantra of "prevention." Disease prevention represents the most perfect strategic practice of medicine, and personal coding is the most important key to effective prevention. Constitutional awareness zeroes in on intolerances well in advance of any potential acute exposure. This is also true for chronic disease. The day-to-day dietary intake of allergenic and intolerance foods contributes to chronic inflammation.

I have designed constitutional health programs for tens of thousands of people with remarkable and consistently replicable results and continue to allay their worries about which foods are good for them. Most of them come in dazed and confused because one health expert tried to convince them that a food or supplement was good for them, while another said that it was bad for them. Meanwhile their doctor insisted that it did nothing at all.

They are starved for, and deserving of, definitive answers. What's worse, they've been hoodwinked into believing that the conventional establishment has the plan for them, when in fact they're the ones with the answers. In America the health care consumer has been systematically disempowered. The orthodoxy has inculcated them with a victimizing form of codependency.

Natural healing and disease prevention power has always belonged to the patient. Our ancestors were their own physicians. They were fully aware of exactly who they were and what they could eat, drink, and do. This ancestral self-awareness represents not only who they were, it reminds us of who we truly are.

CONSTITUTION CODING, PAST AND PRESENT

Our ancestors had no other choice than to be experts on coding. Their survival depended on their mastery of constitutional awareness. They viewed life from a natural cosmological perspective. To them the universe was a vast whole, comprised of uniquely different parts, and each part was viewed as a separate microuniverse unto itself. Ancient Egyptian, Greek, Roman, Ayurvedic, and Arabic cultures adopted detailed constitutional systems for their well-being and the advancement of their civilizations.

Every ancient culture established a system whereby they cosmologically linked themselves with the natural world in an elemental fashion. That is, they classified different types of human personality types as, say, fire, earth, air, or water. Fire may have been chosen to represent a person with a fiery personality. Air might represent someone inclined to deep, pensive thought. These elemental systems provided them with the means to better understand the uniqueness of each person's constitution, further enabling them to correct energy imbalances that might otherwise result in dis-ease.

Constitution refers to one's general state of health in accordance with the individual's unique tendencies, and is believed to be closely related to pathogenesis. It reflects the overall state of body, mind, and spirit. It is a concept related to physiology, psychology, temperament, and behavior. The system employed by the ancient Japanese was called *godai*, and it established the symbols of air, water, ether, fire, and the void to refer to their five different constitutions. The Tibetans established their Bon system of air, water, earth, ether, and fire. The ancient Babylonians differentiated their constitutional types as earth, fire, sky, wind, and sea. The alchemy of medieval and Renaissance Europe was a bit more complex, with an eight-element constitutional concept of air, water, ether, fire, earth, mercury, sulfur, and salt. The ancient Greeks had their four humors, the Hindus their *Tatta* system, and the Buddhists established a constitutional concept called *Mahābhūta*.

The one thing these systems all had in common was their intention to establish a deeper understanding of the energetic uniqueness of each and every person in context with an infinite cosmos of energy. They appreciated that life force defined everything and that everything projected its own personal expression of life force. Moreover, they knew that, when properly deciphered, constitution coding could assist in the maintaining of a balanced life.

According to the system of classical Chinese medicine, there is a detailed constitutional theory called the Five Elements Principle. This system first establishes that there are two primary health-related constitutions: 1) congenital and 2) acquired.

Congenital constitution refers to the general state of health and tendencies a child inherits from her parents. Congenital constitution is thought of as the essence (which in today's terms we would call DNA) that a child is born with. Whole Health teaches that the congenital constitution represents our "fixed code," the unique and unalterable aspects of who we are.

Acquired constitution refers to the changing influences that arise from nourishment, lifestyle, and general day-to-day living.

The foods we eat, the thoughts we think, the love and lifestyle we cultivate, all play a significant role in balancing the influences of our congenital constitution. Acquired constitution represents what Whole Health calls our "mutable code."

One of the fundamental beliefs of Chinese medicine is that human beings are infinitely intertwined with all of nature. The ancient Chinese classified all of nature into a handful of basic elements.

They mapped out five energetic classifications intended to represent the unique distinctions between everything in nature. They divided the entire multiverse of unseen energy into five separate categories for the purposes of establishing unique distinctions and dynamic contrasts. Here they could plainly distinguish the differences and similarities between all things. They understood that in order to prosper, live, adapt, and survive, they would need to better understand the uniqueness of the energies within the mosaic of life.

To their way of thinking, the universe was comprised of varying energies that constantly required balancing. This concept was applied directly in their practice of medicine and disease prevention. Balancing your energy would require different foods and medicines than your neighbor would. These constitutional prescriptions would also have to change seasonally, in accordance with the fluidity of nature. What you ate, drank, and took medicinally was constantly changing, as the seasons brought forth their respective energetic cycles. There is no one-size-fits-all approach to living—and it is dynamic, not static. They didn't all eat the same wheat, drink the same milk, or take Lipitor forever. Everyone's needs, tendencies, and behaviors were respected and treated in accordance with their ever-changing individual needs.

Each of the five element classifications is associated with a graphic symbol to represent what are believed to be the primary categories of all and everything that exists between heaven and earth. The origins of these five energy distinctions are quite logical, when you think about it.

THE FIVE MANIFESTATIONS OF ENERGY

1. Abundance
2. Excess
3. Balance
4. Deficiency
5. Insufficiency

To the ancients, the universe was a dynamic domain of living change driven by a powerful, unseen life force. They envisioned the circuiting heavens, the changing seasons, the wind, rain, snow, and every living being as an embodiment of one of the five manifestations of energy. In energy terms, everything either had an abundance, excess, balance, deficiency, or an insufficiency of life force. They understood the vital importance of distinguishing the differences between all energies, so they devised a system with five metaphors that represented the energy differences for all dynamic energies. These became known as the five constitutional elements.

THE FIVE CONSTITUTION CODES (FIXED)

1. Wood—abundant energy
2. Fire—excess energy
3. Earth—balanced energy
4. Metal—deficient energy
5. Water—insufficient energy

Remember, the five classifications of elements pertained to everything in the universe, including you and me. We all fit somewhere within those five elements.

Within the extended cosmological tapestry of the Five Elements Principle, the ancient Chinese established five metaphors to align with each unique constitutional type. Your first step to Whole Health is deciphering your fixed constitution code. This exercise is Whole Health's attempt to bring each reader to a closer appreciation of their constitutional uniqueness. The following chapters deal more specifically with mutable constitution codes and muscle testing. This is where Whole Health truly distinguishes itself as a system that enables its practitioners to tune in to the specific changing needs of every individual. Where the constitution codes break each of us down into five separate types, Whole Health reveals the uniqueness of each and every one of us in a dynamic, ever-changing way. It all begins with constitution.

DECIPHERING YOUR FIXED CONSTITUTION CODE

Deciphering your fixed constitution code is an extremely important step to becoming your own self-empowered Whole Health–care manager. Remember, we all have *fixed constitution codes*, which never change, and *mutable constitution codes*, which are forever changing. The questionnaire below will help you to determine your fixed constitution code only. (The chapters that follow will guide you through the process of deciphering and working with your mutable code.)

Whole Health has distilled its constitutional decoding process down to fifteen central questions. These fifteen questions represent the keys to unlocking the door to your fixed constitution code. For each category, select the letter corresponding to the response that BEST describes you. *Note:* For questions 1 and 4, please respond with an answer that best describes you **during your formative and early adult years**, even though you may no longer entirely fit that description.

1. **BODY TYPE** (*in early adulthood*) _____
   a. Strong, well-defined
   b. Soft, round
   c. Medium
   d. Medium, lean
   e. Thin, lean

2. **STAMINA** _____
   a. Good energy, good endurance
   b. High energy, poor endurance
   c. Moderate energy, inconsistent endurance
   d. Low energy, always conserves
   e. Very low energy, physically inactive

3. **HEALTH VULNERABILITY** _____
   a. Liver/digestive
   b. Heart/stress
   c. Spleen/general immune
   d. Lung/allergy
   e. Genito-urinary/hormonal/skeletal

4. **POSITIVE MENTAL NATURE** (*at your best*) _____
   a. Confident, independent
   b. Enthusiastic, exciting
   c. Nurturing, caring
   d. Logical, precise
   e. Cautious, conservative

5. **NEGATIVE MENTAL NATURE** (*at your worst*) _____
   a. Obstinate, argumentative
   b. Impulsive, consuming
   c. Meddlesome, manipulative
   d. Obsessive, perfectionistic
   e. Stagnant, withdrawn

6. **POSITIVE EMOTIONAL NATURE** (*at your best*) _____
   a. Kind, giving
   b. Joyous, optimistic
   c. Compassionate, warm
   d. Courageous, bold
   e. Calm, peaceful

7. **NEGATIVE EMOTIONAL NATURE** (*at your worst*) _____
   a. Angry, impatient
   b. Vengeful, impulsive
   c. Anxious, dysfunctional
   d. Melancholic, depressed
   e. Fearful, disassociated

8. **SPIRITUAL TENDENCY** _____
   a. Agnostic
   b. Mystical
   c. Pantheistic
   d. Orthodox
   e. Unorthodox

9. **YOUR PERSONA IN YOUR FAMILY RELATIONSHIPS** _____
   a. Performer
   b. Idealist
   c. Peacemaker
   d. Perfectionist
   e. Escapist

10. **YOUR PERSONA IN YOUR ROMANTIC RELATIONSHIPS** _____
    a. Loyal
    b. Tempestuous

   c. Warm

   d. Detached

   e. Mysterious

11. SEXUAL NATURE _____

   a. Passionate

   b. Magnetic

   c. Passive

   d. Dispassionate

   e. Erotic

12. YOUR PERSONA UNDER STRESS _____

   a. Persistent

   b. Burned out

   c. Escapist

   d. Intellectual

   e. Avoidant

13. NATURAL AFFINITY _____

   a. To be independent

   b. To feel pleasure

   c. To feel secure

   d. To have order

   e. To be left alone

14. BASIC INSTINCT _____

   a. To assert

   b. To attract

   c. To nurture

   d. To organize

   e. To continue

15. **LIFE'S PURPOSE** _____
- **a.** To make an impact
- **b.** To be loved
- **c.** To make peace
- **d.** To systematize
- **e.** To learn and teach

Total Responses for A _____ **B** _____ **C** _____ **D** _____ **E** _____

Now look at your total for each category. What is the lettered category (A, B, C, D, or E) with the highest total? The letters correspond to the constitutional types below, so if the category with the highest total is A, then you have a Wood constitution. If the highest total is B, then you have a Fire constitution, and so on.

A. Wood
B. Fire
C. Earth
D. Metal
E. Water

We all reflect a combination of code tendencies. The goal of this questionnaire is merely to help you identify your *Fixed Constitution code*.

In the next chapter you will begin to learn the Whole Health system of Electromagnetic Muscle Testing (EMT). This will enable you to maximize your Whole Health by teaching you to identify and adapt to your ever-changing mutable code.

THE DETAILS OF YOUR FIXED CONSTITUTION CODE

1. Wood Constitution

General Constitution: Wood types are impulsive, exciting, and active. They have great strength and conviction and you always know right where they stand. They make honest, true, and loyal friends and partners. Above all else, they are reliable and can be counted on even when the odds are not favorable. Woods must be careful with their tendency to overcommit, however, as they tend to get depleted with all they take on. Woods know no other way but to work until they drop! Wood types should be wary of partnering up with Fire and Metal types, as these are very likely to drain their precious energy. Woods do best with Water types, who are inclined to nurture and replenish them.

Physical (early adult years): Woods are typically defined by a squarely built, well-defined frame. They tend to be of average weight and are rarely overweight. Their complexion is slightly oily, thick, and ruddy. Their hair is dark brown and coarse. Their eyes are usually green, blue-green, or hazel. They tend to have a very strong appetite and are frequently troubled by constipation. Woods have good energy and good endurance with a resting pulse that's quick and vibrant (70–80 beats per minute), but they're very light sleepers. Wood types are a passionate breed with good sexual stamina.

Mental/Emotional/Spiritual: When at their best mentally, Woods are confident and independent—emotionally they're kind and giving. Spiritually they are often agnostic. Wood types are generally high-performance, loyal, persistent, independent, and assertive. They are Spartans who have a knack for making an impact, but they can be intimidating.

Health Problems: Woods are often bloated, gassy with a distended abdomen after eating. They tend to have poor dietary discrimination, crave fatty foods, and suffer from acne, dry burning eyes, muscle cramps, tendinitis, labile hypertension, gallstones, conjunctivitis, hepatitis, glaucoma, Ménière's disease, hormonal imbalances, earaches, impulsive behavior, shingles, mood swings, light sensitivity, blurred vision, cysts, jaundice, myasthenia gravis, gout, and alcoholism.

Balancing Diet: Sour foods are best for wood types, as sour helps their body to gather up energy. The list of strengthening sour foods for Wood types includes nonfermented soy products, barley, Brussels sprouts, cabbage, kohlrabi, leeks, scallions, and most fruits.

Balancing Herbs: Achyranthes, barberry, campsis, chaenomeles, crataegus (hawthorn), elderberry, *Fructus corni* (dogwood), *Fructus mume* (black plum), rose hips from *Rosa laevigatae* (Cherokee rose), the fruit of *Schisandra chinensis,* grapefruit seed extract, hawthorn berry, Oregon grape root, peony, and rose hips.

Balancing Nutritional Supplements: Homeopathic natrum sulphuricum, hepar sulphuricum, lycopodium, choline, lecithin, and methionine.

2. *Fire Constitution*

General Constitution: Fire types are extremely overactive. They tend to be active even when they are doing nothing. They are distracted, fidgety, and are constantly moving on to the next thing. Fires are intensely passionate, but because they burn so bright, they must be very careful not to burn out. They are inspiring and charismatic, and everything seems to stand still when they enter the room. They have the gift to excite and are themselves very excitable. Fires can vacillate between being magnetic and repellent, as they can be overstimulating at times. There is no middle ground with Fires— Fires are all or nothing. They do best in partnerships with Wood and Earth types but must be careful not to exhaust them. Fires must avoid Water types, as they are inclined to put out their fire.

Physical (early adult years): Fire types tend to have a medium to fuller frame. Their complexion is oily, with a burned brown tint and red cheeks. Their hair tends to be red or brown. Their eyes are often dark brown. They tend to have a constant and strong appetite and their bowels are normal, with occasional constipation when under stress. They have high energy and poor endurance with a resting pulse that's fast (80+ bpm) and irregular. When it comes to sleep, they tend to be insomniacs. Sexually they are often magnetic and tempestuous. Under duress they have a tendency to burn out.

Mental/Emotional/Spiritual: When feeling positive, Fires are enthusiastic and exciting as well as joyous and optimistic. When feeling afflicted, they are impulsive, consuming, and often vengeful. Spiritually they often project a powerful, mystical quality. The Fire type has a tendency toward idealism. They are pleasure-seekers who often get bored very easily. Their natural instinct is to attract. Fires are charismatic, self-concerned, and need constant love and approval.

Health Problems: Fire types often have a tendency toward heartburn. They eat too fast, get hot and sweaty after eating, crave foods constantly, and have red, burning ears. They often suffer from fever blisters on the tongue, varicose veins, rheumatoid arthritis, essential hypertension, Raynaud's disease, heart arrhythmias, hyperthyroidism, Parkinson's disease, multiple sclerosis, hot flashes, mastitis, nervous conditions, fainting spells, hypoglycemia, low blood pressure, acidosis, cerebral palsy, hyperactivity, phlebitis, tremors, day sweats, blood clots, hypochondria, and angina.

Balancing Diet: Fire types are ideally suited energetically for bitter foods. Fires also tend to have an imbalanced excess of energy, which bitter foods release. Examples of balancing bitter foods for Fire types include: shellfish, carrot greens, artichokes, watercress, macadamia nuts, pine nuts, amaranth, quinoa, rye, papaya, olive oil, arugula, asparagus, beet greens, burdock root, daikon radish, dandelion root, kale, romaine lettuce, okra, sprouts, and turnip greens.

Balancing Herbs: Andrographis, barberry root, buplurum root, chaparral, chicory root, chickweed, coptis, echinacea, elecampane, elderflower, gardenia, goldenseal, gotu kola, hawthorn berry, honeysuckle, magnolia flower, milk thistle, myrrh, wild gooseberry, and yellow dock.

Balancing Nutritional Supplements: Omega-3 fish oils, flaxseeds, ubiquinol, GPLC, magnesium asporotate, ace peptides, menaquinone, and serrapeptase.

3. Earth Constitution

General Constitution: Earth types are givers, nurturers, and peacemakers. They make the world feel welcomed, cared for, and loved. Regardless of whether they are male or female, Earths all have a mothering quality about them. The problem is they not only give, they give in—they can't seem to say no. Earth types rarely get enough back in return from others, and they tend to ignore their own needs as well. Earth types are not enamored of the latest fashion trends. They're down-home types with a focus on comfort and grounding. They love their homes and are always at their best there. They love raising children and nurturing their mate in every way. They are inclined to intermittent periods of depression and anxiety. If unhappy, they are also inclined to sugar, carbohydrate, and alcohol addictions. They are built for comfort and will seek it to the extreme if stressed. Earths are best suited for partnerships with Fire types and should try to avoid Woods.

Physical (early adult years): Earth types are generally characterized by a broad frame that is typically overweight. Their complexion is smooth, sensitive, well hydrated, and apricot-tinted. They're inclined to have medium brown hair with medium texture, and medium brown eyes. They have a moderate appetite at mealtime and a bigger appetite for dessert. Their elimination tends to be normal to slightly loose under stress. They have moderate energy but erratic endurance. Their pulse tends to be moderate and even (60–70 bpm). They are sound sleepers and have a high requirement for sleep. Sexually they tend to be somewhat passive, but are very affectionate.

Mental/Emotional/Spiritual: When feeling positive, Earths are supportive and caring. When feeling afflicted, they tend to be meddlesome and manipulative. Emotionally they are often spiritually pantheistic. They are peacemakers with little stamina for conflict. They have a strong need for security and very much dislike having to adapt to change. Their basic instinct is to be caring and nurturing. Their life's purpose is to heal and make peace. They are mediators who are susceptible to manipulation.

Health Problems: Those with Earth constitutions are prone to chronic phlegmatic conditions. They often suffer from sugar and starch addictions. They tend to suffer from bloat, bloody gums, fever blisters, stiff aching muscles, fibromyalgia, colitis, gastric ulcers, chronic fatigue, enteritis, anemia, low thyroid, hemorhoids, diabetes, nausea, parasitosis, athlete's foot, chronic candidiasis, Lyme disease, pancreatic insufficiency, mononucleosis, anal fissures, encephalopathy, Hodgkin's disease, and retroviruses.

Balancing Diet: The diet best suited for the Earth type is a sweet-flavor diet, but not too much, as they are prone to addiction. Also, "sweet" has a much broader meaning than usual here; it refers to sustaining proteins as well as root vegetables and natural sweets. Sweet balances and harmonizes the energy of those with an Earth constitution. Sweet foods include all animal proteins, all beans, beets, carrots, corn, peas, potatoes, sweet potatoes, winter squash, yams, almonds, cashews, pumpkin seeds, sesame seeds, sunflower seeds, walnuts, dairy, barley malt, brown rice syrup, stevia, rice, buckwheat, kamut, millet, oats, spelt, teff, triticale, wheat, and all fruits.

Balancing Herbs: Aloe vera, astragalus, basil, chickweed, cinnamon, codonopsis, cordyceps, fenugreek, licorice, lycium, marshmallow, mullein, red clover, *Schisandra chinensis* fruit, Siberian ginseng, and slippery elm.

Balancing Nutritional Supplements: Propolis, chromium, methyl B_{12}, white chestnut (Bach flower remedy), vitamin A, and gamma E.

4. Metal Constitution

General Constitution: Metal types are very exacting people. Everything has to be just right, or else. When it comes to Metal types, cleanliness and order isn't next to godliness, it *is* godliness! They make great managers and community organizers but can easily draw the ire of those closest to them for completely missing out on the deeper meaning of life. Discerning and mathematical, Metals are the world's greatest problem solvers. They must be very careful, however, not to create problems with their obsessive tendency to solve problems. While they make great providers, they are often criticized for lacking warmth and passion—that is, until they become saddened by the recognition of all the preciousness they've missed out on in life. Then they tend to become so grief-stricken and depressed that they are difficult to tolerate. Metals are wise to avoid commitments with Fire types and are best partnered with the Earth constitution.

Physical (early adult years): The Metal type is generally erect with a medium build. They tend to be ten pounds or more underweight. Their complexion is smooth, sensitive, well hydrated, and with an apricot tint. Their hair is medium blond, platinum, white, or light brown, and of very fine texture. Their eyes are pale blue or light brown. Their appetite is light to moderate. Their bowel movements tend to vacillate between constipation and diarrhea. They have low energy and poor endurance, and their resting pulse is slow and deep (50–60 bpm). They are deep sleepers but have no difficulty waking.

Mental/Emotional/Spiritual: Metals are logical and precise and can be obsessive and ritualistic. When they feel positive, they are courageous and bold. When they feel afflicted, they are melancholic. Spiritually they tend to be orthodox. Sexually they are mechanistic and can be dispassionate. They are inclined to be perfectionistic and detached, and are given to overintellectualization. They crave order and don't do well with spontaneity. They love to organize and implement systems. Their perfectionism is their most negative trait.

Health Problems: Metal types tend to suffer from bedsores, loss of the sense of smell, asthma, bronchitis, emphysema, sinus infections, allergies, cystic fibrosis, dehydration, nasal polyps, sore throats, strep throat, tracheitis, tonsillitis, pharyngitis, mastoiditis, tuberculosis, chronically inflamed adenoids, appendicitis, Crohn's disease, and irritable bowel syndrome.

Balancing Diet: Metals require pungent (spicy) foods to disperse and balance their energy. These include sardines, bok choy, currants, garlic, ginger, leeks, mustard greens, onions, parsley, parsnips, peppers, radish, scallions, and turnips,

Balancing Herbs: Angelica, arugula, anise, basil, cayenne pepper, chrysanthemum, cinnamon, *Concha ostreae*, coriander, fenugreek, ginger, magnolia flower, mint, mullein, myrrh, os draconis, pepper, skullcap, spearmint, turmeric, and yarrow.

Balancing Nutritional Supplements: Gorse (Bach flower remedy), NAC, homeopathic *Spongia tosta*, vitamin A, and vitamin D.

5. Water Constitution

General Constitution: Water types are deep, reflective thinkers. They like to while away the hours reminiscing and contemplating, and are very inclined to meditation and visualization. They make good spiritual students and teachers, mystics, intuitives, and quantum physicists. They are innately inclined to comprehend the deeper meaning of life and are capable of communicating it to others with ease. They may tend to become so reclusive that they become loners. They also have an affinity for losing track of reality as they become too wrapped up in the world within their mind. Water types are best matched with Metal types but they must try to avoid long-term relationships with Earth types.

Physical (early adult years): Water types have a small, thin frame. They range from average weight to five pounds underweight. Their complexion is cold, clammy, pale, and white. Their eyes are dark blue. They have little or no appetite and tend to contend with frequent diarrhea. They have very low energy and poor endurance. Their resting pulse is very low (40–50 bpm) and shallow. In many cases their sleep is disturbed by frequent urination.

Mental/Emotional/Spiritual: When feeling positive, Waters are cautious, conservative, and have great wisdom. They are also calm and peaceful under ideal circumstances. When feeling afflicted, they are overcome with irrational fears and tend to become disassociated. Spiritually they are unorthodox. Sexually they are often drawn to eroticism. They are mysterious escapists who deeply reflect. They like to be left alone, and hate being exposed. They always persevere. They evince a certain genius and they make exceptional teachers. Their archetype is the recluse.

Health Problems: Water types show little interest in food. They often feel faint after eating, crave salt, have dark circles under the eyes, suffer hearing loss, and have chronic lower-back pain. They often suffer from osteoporosis, kidney stones, cystitis, edema, urinary tract infections, lupus, nephritis, sexual infertility/impotence, urinary incontinence, memory loss, insomnia, night sweats, sensory and motor problems, alkalosis, enuresis, syphilis, anorexia, gonorrhea, scoliosis, mercury poisoning, agoraphobia, and bulimia.

Balancing Diet: Salty foods tend to soften, moisten, and balance the kidneys and adrenal glands of the Water type. Among the best examples of balancing salty foods are sea bass, pinto beans, chestnuts, endive, escarole, Bibb lettuce, Concord grapes, olives, seaweed, sorrel, spinach, and Swiss chard.

Balancing Herbs: Actinolite, cassia, cistanche, clematis, isatis leaf, parsley, red clover, rehmannia, sargassum, scrophularia, kunbu, and natrii sulfas.

Balancing Nutritional Supplements: Cranberry capsules, mimulus (Bach flower remedy), homeopathic *Eupatorium purpureum*, zinc gluconate, and raw kidney tablets.

CODE COMPATIBILITY

It is important to note that many of the foods and herbs mentioned in the above discussion of "types" generate more than one flavor, and may therefore occupy multiple categories. Each code type energetically affects and is affected by all other code types. Some codes will tend to have a positive influence, while others will tend to have a negative effect on each other. To understand these interconnections, we must perform "code compatibility." When constitutional types are compatibly matched, relationships are very likely to flourish.

Most Compatible Constitutional Matches

1. Woods energize Fires
2. Fires energize Earths
3. Earths energize Metals
4. Metals energize Waters
5. Waters energize Woods

Least Compatible Constitutional Matches

1. Woods deplete Earths
2. Earths deplete Waters
3. Waters deplete Fires
4. Fires deplete Metals
5. Metals deplete Woods

You have initiated the process of identifying your unique energetic identity. In the chapters that follow, Whole Health will teach you to decipher, balance, and adapt to your ever-changing mutable nature, instructing you in how to detail your own constitutional wellness program. You will then be able to create the diet and lifestyle best suited to your specific, ever-changing energy needs.

CHAPTER 3

SIXTH-SENSORY ENERGY DIAGNOSIS

THE SIXTH SENSE

Before presenting the complete Whole Health energy system of assessing, balancing, and preserving mutable constitutionality, I would first like to eradicate some age-old, sixth-sensory barriers and invite readers, with open arms, into a realm of higher possibility.

The Whole Health system of energy diagnosis is based on unconventional sixth-sensory techniques. Ours is a five-sensory, material culture and, to date, most sixth-sensory arguments have only served to marginalize themselves with their lack of gravity. Thus, though there remains a great divide as to the real plausibility of sixth-sensory applications, and though it is rarely presented in a convincing intellectual manner, sixth-sensory reality is undeniable. The evidence is everywhere.

Following the great South Asian tsunami of 2004, scientists

were drawn to reports of aboriginal tribesmen who exhibited extra-sensory anticipation of the disaster well before it happened, affording them time to escape to higher ground. A number of recent studies have advanced new theories that the brain's anterior cingulate cortex has the ability to function as an intuitive early warning system. Scientists have established that the anterior cingulate cortex and the subconscious mind work together to anticipate life events before they actually happen, without our being consciously aware of it. But ongoing research has, of late, begun discovering multiple areas of brain involvement in sixth-sensory awareness. A mosaic of brain and mind energies work as convergent forces, coming together to create a mystical realm of higher possibility, and science is beginning to pay attention.

When NASA Jet Propulsion Laboratory scientists lost communication with their Mars Polar Lander space probe as it entered the red planet's atmosphere in 1999, the result was a devastating $4 million loss. The project's managers were forced to find viable solutions for anticipating and avoiding the future prospects of additional costly errors. They immediately assembled an expert research team to begin studying how the brain tracks down and processes its own errors through a mechanism called error-related negativity (ERN).

ERN is an electromagnetic voltage wave phenomenon that activates beneath the skull near the midbrain. This wave is triggered by the neurotransmitter dopamine, and is measurable whenever the brain detects error. Following the ERN wave, the brain stops producing dopamine, which activates the basal ganglia and (emotional) limbic system. There is also activation within the deeper cortex that sends signals to executive brain areas to correct error before it happens. In short, error-related negativity is a neurobiological mind-brain phenomenon that actually triggers alert signals prior to error. Voltage is said to decline by 10 microvolts approximately 100 milliseconds prior to an error event. The scientific community isn't the only establishment group that's beginning to acknowledge that we are naturally wired for both sensory and extrasensory awareness.

In February 2012, the U.S. Office of Naval Research posted a notice that the U.S. Navy was intent on developing sixth-sense research. In the notice, they expressed that existing research has proven that humans are capable of detecting and acting in unique patterns without intellectual analysis. The U.S. Army has also conducted studies suggesting that a sixth sense can arise from implicit learning—the absorption of information without an awareness of the learning process. The army is currently designing sixth-sensory virtual battlefield training programs.

Legendary psychotherapist Carl Jung often spoke of intuitive types as acting not upon rational judgment, but rather from sheer intensity of perception. The great Conrad Hilton of Hilton Hotels fame was said to have had intuitive dreams that tipped him off as to the exact amount of money he should offer on his property bids. During one of his most important property deals, he was said to have prepared to bid no more than $165,000 for the property. The night before all bids were to be in, a dream clearly instructed him to bid exactly $180,000, which he did. He eventually secured the property, and it ultimately garnered him more than $2 million in profit. Hilton later discovered that the next highest bid was $179,800.

Historical accounts tell us that ten days prior to his assassination, Abraham Lincoln had a dream that the entire nation was passing through the East Wing of the White House, grieving the death of the president. On July 22, 1961, President John F. Kennedy wrote a note revealing a premonition of his untimely death on November 22, 1963: he'd been told by God that a place had been made for him, and that he would soon be coming to take his rest.

Many of us have had experiences where we've correctly anticipated events well in advance of their happening. I will never forget an interesting, intuitive experience that I had at the age of twelve. I was driving with my mother from our home in upstate New York to visit my brother, who was living in Lynn, Massachusetts. As I looked out of the car window at the world going by, I fixed my gaze and suddenly went into a trance state. I remember going deep into my mind to some very deep, faraway place. As I did I had a series of remarkable visions of my own future. I clearly saw that I would live in Massachusetts and that I would be a very different kind of doctor who would help a great many people. I also saw that I would have two sons and one daughter. I conveyed this to my mother, who simply replied, "That's good, Mark." Little did she know that all my visions would come to pass.

My dear dad was abruptly awakened by a premonition on what turned out to be his last day on Earth. My stepmother tells of how he rose up startled in the middle of the night following a dream he'd had of himself hanging in the woods. The next morning he went off to clear some wooded property that he'd just purchased. After just a few hours of working in those woods, his heart stopped. It seems as though a sixth-sensory premonition had projected through my father's last dream on Earth.

When it comes to sixth-sensory consciousness, there are a myriad of important questions that might be considered, as we are clearly dealing with a remarkable phenomenon. Being who I am, my questions were always about whether we could ever harness sixth-sensory power to heal. I often wondered: Can sixth-sensory awareness manifest as a collective consciousness, and can it be perceived at nonlocal distances? What predisposes one to arouse such an uncommon sense, and can it be commanded? Some of the scientific answers I had always hoped for have at last begun to surface.

Researcher Trish Stafford, neuropsychotherapist at the University of Technology in Sydney, Australia, recently led a study of 30 volunteers aged 21 to 65 who were evaluated for 180 hours, hooked up to electrocardiographs, and monitored for skin conductance resonance to help identify what is described as a "heightened moment of awareness." Stafford discovered that the subjects' nervous systems could be aligned or unified in sync, despite having no physical contact with one another. This study was peer reviewed in four journals, and is considered to be the first of its kind to have discovered that when the brain's parietal lobe is triggered into action, a sixth sense is engaged.

Respected Cornell University psychologist Daryl Bem has conducted sixth-sensory precognition studies with more than 1,000 volunteers and submitted his findings to peer-reviewed scientific journals. In one study, he asked volunteers to view a computer screen with two curtains. He asked the volunteers to guess which curtain had a randomly placed, computerized erotic photo behind it. The subjects guessed correctly 53 percent of the time. Moreover, Bem noted that subjects' physiological arousal responses to the erotic photos occurred a full two to three seconds prior to the actual appearance of the photograph. In short, arousal appears to influence sixth-sensory awareness.

The Princeton Engineering Anomalies Research (PEAR) program represents nearly three decades of scientific human consciousness studies. The PEAR lab was founded by former dean of engineering Robert G. Jahn. Jahn proposed trials to measure whether or not collective human consciousness could be traced with highly sensitive electronic devices. To do so, he and his team constructed what they called the Random Event Generator (REG), a finely tuned sensory receptor that could pick up changes and peaks in human energy. PEAR researchers hypothesized that there was a collective consciousness that generated a strong enough field of energy to be traced by the REG. The researchers were able to track changes in collective human energy transmissions, especially during holidays such as Christmas and New Year's Eve. Just prior to the attacks on September 11, 2001, REGs were placed at virtually every corner of the globe while still being linked to the master computer in Princeton. The strongest peak in human collective consciousness readings was reported a full two to three hours prior to the World Trade Center disaster, seeming to indicate that a collective sixth sense was engaged in anticipation of the tragedy.

Ready or not, sixth-sensory medicine has gone mainstream. Northwestern University recently introduced a remarkable, innovative program with their newly developed Raby Institute for Integrative Medicine. The institute offers an array of intuitive and energy-healing programs, including healing touch, body talk, bio-electromagnetic therapy, Reiki, Qigong, and other vibrational medicine modalities. Their approach places a great emphasis on innate emotion and unconscious intuition as a means to guide patients to better health.

The emergence of programs such as the Raby Institute signals a radical shift in the way we're approaching health care in America. There is growing interest in energy and sixth-sensory approaches to healing that are now becoming a part of the mainstream landscape.

Sixth-sensory awareness is nothing more than a reservoir of inner knowing that operates from deep within the recesses of our unconscious minds. It's merely been excluded from the picture of our everyday reality. The Buddhists refer to "no mind," a purer stream of consciousness that eradicates the clumsiness of cognitive processes. It's a little like the martial arts philosophy of karate, which means "empty hand." The more you empty out your own force, the more the emptiness allows for a greater force to take over.

The debate rages on as to whether or not sixth-sensory awareness can be consistently and reliably tapped into. Is it a pipe dream, or is it just that we've been programmed to think of it as such? Can a materially biased culture such as ours harness sixth-sensory awareness in ways that enhance our lifestyle, health, and healing?

Noted American theoretical physicist Dr. David Bohm frequently addressed the concept of sixth-sensory inner knowing from a quantum perspective. He theorized that there was an upper-dimensional space, a field rife with the flow of infinite information, and that the energy generated by the vacuum of its fluctuations provided a background illumination for our ordinary world.

Thus, to Bohm's way of thinking, sixth-sensory awareness is the illuminating of our ordinary world of possibilities, which taps into the quantum field of infinite information. In other words, reductionist thinking isn't likely to access it, and it's not energy that's going to announce itself to us. The quantum sixth-sensory field of infinite information that Bohm refers to requires expansionist thinking open to discovery. The quantum sixth-sensory field has the potential of shedding a light of infinite possibilities on our ordinary world.

SIXTH-SENSORY DIAGNOSIS

At the energy level, we are forever shifting and changing. A food that you healthfully consumed yesterday may produce a mild headache today. You might need a break from a friend you've been spending a great deal of time with. Whole Health Healing has developed detailed systems to help you keep up with your mutable energy needs. Adapting to your subtle energy needs will further enable you to keep all your vital energies in balance. When your energies are in balance, your whole being is better in balance. Let me explain the Whole Health system sixth-sensory muscle-testing system that I developed.

There are many systems of muscle testing and as many theories about how and why it works. Whole Health has developed its own muscle-testing system as a medium for sixth-sensory diagnosis. The system is called Electromagnetic Muscle Testing (EMT). The term *ch'i,* or *life force,* reveals a great deal about why this muscle-testing system is so effective. All living humans emit an electromagnetic energy, or "life force," and modern medicine routinely performs MRIs, EEGs, and EKGs—tests that measure human bioelectricity in the body, brain, and heart. This imbuing energy represents the quintessential life force, the difference between living and nonliving bodies, a balance of which is synonymous with vibrant health.

Scottish researcher Dr. Rutger Wever, who was once an associate of Max Planck's at the Institute for Behavioral Psychology, tells us that human bioelectricity transmits approximately 0.025 volts of ambient electrical charge. We know that the heart pumps electricity, and that the brain stores and redistributes it at somewhere between 3 and 50 cycles per second (Hz).

Human bioelectricity is synonymous with the nervous system (neurology). Our nervous system is our electrical system. We react automatically at this neurological level continuously from moment to moment, without ever being aware of it.

Let's look at this system in action. Say you're having a bad dream, and in this dream you're being chased. Your neurological response generates an elevated heart rate, elevated blood pressure, and perspiration. Yes, you can produce all of these very real biological responses from a mere dream state, triggered by stimuli that aren't even real! You need only imagine or recall a potentially threatening event to set off these highly sensitive neural triggers, but there is much more than fundamental biology at work here.

Within our bodies there is a constant flow of communication taking place from cell to cell, first triggered by the heart. There is a bundle of afferent nerves (sensory receptors) in the heart called the cardiac intrinsic ganglia (the little brain within the heart) that first receive the messages from the mind that determine the degree of safety or threat posed by any given stimuli. The cardiac intrinsic ganglia then relay the message to the big brain, which in turn transmits it to the nervous system. Once the nervous system gets the "thumbs-up" or "thumbs-down" on the safety assessment, it then conveys the message to every cell in the body.

Regardless of whether you are having a bad dream, listening to a negative conversation, remembering a hurtful event, watching a boxing match or old news footage of 9/11, you are going to activate your mind to heart, your heart to brain, and brain to nervous system in a biofeedback loop. Nature designed our biofeedback loop to be a failsafe system because survival of our species was clearly the ultimate priority.

Our all-important survival communication system begins with superconscious, extrasensory awareness about what is good for us and what is bad for us. It is a rapid-fire, pass/fail assessment system that judges potential stimuli as welcome or unwelcome in our world, and the reactions are universal only to a point. We all generate warning signals when confronted by potential threats, but what of more mundane stimuli? Remember that this biofeedback loop activates for absolutely everything that enters into our field of perception. What then of dairy or wheat? What about your dog's hair or the pollen from the grass in your front yard? These all represent exposures that generate a response from your biofeedback system. Where an attack by a wild animal in the woods will prompt the same negative nerve feedback for nearly all of us, only some of us exhibit a negative reaction to dairy, wheat, pollen, and so on. This reveals two very important things: First, the biofeedback loop is a very reliable system designed as a priority survival system by nature. Second, it helps us to gain access to and adapt to the needs of our mutable constitution. At this subtle energy level, we all react very uniquely to more than half of the potential stimuli we are confronted with.

Our nervous system is an extended network of nerve endings and nerve pathways, like a telecommunications grid system that runs through the entire body. Because it runs through all of the muscles, whenever we are asked about or confronted with anything, our brain initiates a communication response to the body throughout the entire nerve network, ultimately talking to the muscles.

The science of psychoneuroimmunology has mapped out this messaging sequence. As the stimuli (dream, stress, food, a question, etc.) enter into your mind and brain's field of awareness, an immediate sensory "sizing-up" process is engaged.

The first brain stop on this journey is a ping-ponging of thought volley between your emotional centers in the amygdala and the hippocampus. Here is where your brain is trying to emotionally sense whether or not the stimuli feel safe.

The next stop is the prefrontal cortex. Here is where your brain settles down to some good old-fashioned logic. After both centers have had their say, a final decision is made. If your mind/heart feels unsafe, things are directed back to anxiety ping-pong until it is determined that you're out of danger. If things are okay, the prefrontal cortex helps to organize your thoughts and stabilize your entire system.

Keep in mind that while all this communication is taking place, your muscles remain the most responsive nerve medium. All stimuli are reacted to and interpreted as safe or unsafe, positive or negative. The earliest detection response is muscular, because muscles activate fight and flight. Simply stated, whenever you feel safe, happy, and positive, the brain sends a *steady, even flow* of neural electricity to your muscles, giving them an abundance of controlled strength. Whenever you feel unsafe, anxious, and negative, the brain sends a highly charged nervous flow of electricity to the muscles, greatly reducing *controlled* strength.

Communication between the body and mind, or *in* the body/ mind, if you will, is constant and the muscles remain the perfect biofeedback system. Try this simple experiment: Ask a friend to simply lift up his arm and resist your attempt to gently push it down. Now ask him to close his eyes and to continue to resist your efforts as you call out contrasting words and images. Compare his resistance responses to words such as *love* versus *hate*, *warmth* versus *cold, fun* versus *boredom,* and *joy* versus *agony.* Next, call out a dozen or so foods and see how the responses vary. You will be amazed.

Science has understood this complex form of communication since the late 1970s, but has yet to be convinced that it can be consistently trusted. When I began my practice, in 1982, I was determined to find out just how trustworthy this communication process was. The theoretical debates continue to this day. Those with a mechanistic bias will never believe, but those with a more vitalistic persuasion will never have to be convinced. I thought that it needed development and ongoing testing over time. Now, nearly thirty years and tens of thousands of patient appointments later, I believe that the constant flow of communication in the body/mind is ever trustworthy. I believe it is a perfect biofeedback resource, provided the "listener" knows how to "listen."

Health care can be reduced into two divergent systems: intervention and prevention. If, as the old adage goes, "an ounce of prevention is worth a pound of cure," our present approach to health care in America should be classified as a lightweight in the fight against disease. If we are truly committed to prevention, more reliable early detection and diagnosis methods—made available to everyone—are essential. The key to better early detection and accurate diagnosis is to include and to better equip the patient to be a diagnostic listener. The more we enable the average person to listen at the subtlest energy levels, the better the health of our nation will be.

INTUITIVE NEUROFEEDBACK

We live in a dualistic universe of opposites: yin and yang, male and female, hot and cold, old and young. With that in mind, we might do well to remember that all human beings are dualistic by nature, possessing both a logical and an intuitive mind. Our cultural influence would have us only believe in a five-sensory world of sight, sound, touch, smell, and taste. We tend to overlook the fact that we have access to a sixth sense that enables us to engage our mind at an extrasensory, intuitive level. And while most of us have had experiences with lucid inner knowing, few of us are aware of just how much time our mind tends to spend on such activities.

Hundreds of cognitive studies over the past three decades have confirmed that those human brain processes that occur automatically, without our conscious awareness, constitute most of our mental life.

Consider that the conscious mind can process 2,000 bits of information per second. Pretty impressive until you realize that our unconscious mind can easily process 400 billion bits of information per second! Most of our 300 to 1,000 thoughts per minute come from our unconscious mind, and our unconscious mind is the domain of direct knowledge, immediate insight, and subliminal perception. The question isn't whether these remarkable properties are innate to us. The question is whether or not we can get comfortable with the idea of harnessing their horsepower.

So how might one consistently and reliably tap into a sixth-sensory place of inner knowing? It's really quite simple. Ask your muscles. Sound confusing? Allow me to explain. . . .

When it comes to our unconscious mind's flow of information, it goes something like this: The heart tells the mind, the mind tells the brain, the brain tells the nervous system, the nervous system tells the muscles. The most consistently reliable information system we possess is our nervous system. Our nerves and muscles make up the perfect biofeedback loop. The human nervous system is a highly sensitive alarm system, designed by nature for the survival of a species. If the mind detects trouble, it relays stress signals to the brain. The brain then transmits nerve signals to mobilize the muscles for emergency. If the mind senses safety, it relays nerve signals to the brain that tell the body to relax. The brain then mobilizes the body for efficiency. So I say we have two distinctly different nervous systems: emergency and efficiency. Thus, your unconscious mind sends messages to you through your nervous system and muscles, based on its assessment as to whether things around you are good or bad, safe or unsafe. Moreover, it's wired to do so every waking and sleeping moment of your life. It's what awakens you in a cold sweat with an elevated heart rate following a bad dream. Your biofeedback system never turns off and is therefore ever reliable. Your unconscious mind and nervous system know everything you need to know at all times. And they're always generating positive energy during the good times and negative energy during the bad.

The next question is, how does one learn to dialogue with their all-knowing, unconscious mind via the nervous system? The answer to that question is simple—just ask your sixth-sensory biofeedback system a question. Let your unconscious mind register the question, allow your nervous system to react, and then tug on a muscle. If the muscle is strong (i.e., stays in place when tugged), consider it a positive response. If the muscle is weak (i.e., allows itself to be moved), it's a negative response. Raise your arm and ask someone to give it a tug as they call out the word *wheat*. If your arm is weak, you are likely intolerant to wheat and should consider avoiding it.

Whole Health Energy Diagnostics is based on an intuitive, neuromuscular biofeedback system intended to support natural homeostasis. This system teaches that wellness is a natural state that results from the unobstructed flow of energy to the vital glands and organs of the body. Negative influences such as allergenic foods that are not well tolerated block the flow of this health-giving energy. To restore oneself to a state of wellness, it's important to implement an intuitive neuromuscular biofeedback system to help identify energy blockages and remove them. What is the power source of this remarkable extrasensory awareness?

THE ANATOMICAL HEART OF
OUR SIXTH SENSE

Our way of life here in the modern West is brain-centric. The ancient East is a heart-centric culture. In 1991, HeartMath Institute researcher Dr. J. Andrew Armour discovered the cardiac intrinsic ganglia, or "little brain within the heart," instantly validating centuries-old, heart-centric Chinese wisdom and providing an important bridge between the modern West and the ancient East. He discovered that the heart's electromagnetic field emits 50,000 femtoteslas (standard measurement of a magnetic field), in contrast to the brain's 10,000. He also learned that the amplitude of the heart's electrical field is sixty times greater than the brain's. Furthermore, he found that it envelops every cell in the body, extending even beyond the body outward in all directions into surrounding space. Armour also established that 65 percent of all sensory awareness flows from the heart to the brain. Armour's research and the ongoing research at the institute continues to extend the bridge between East and West.

Between 2004 and 2007, HeartMath researchers performed a number of studies looking at the electrophysiological evidence of intuition, as well as precognition studies on serial entrepreneurial intuition. They've consistently discovered that the body appears to receive and respond to emotionally charged stimuli a full six to eight seconds before events are actually experienced. Once again, the heart appears to be the place of origin where intuition is operated. The researchers consistently note a higher heart rate recorded prior to the event that would cause said increase.

Similarly, a September 2012 study published in the journal *Proceedings of the National Academy of Sciences* and performed by researchers from Massachusetts General Hospital, Beth Israel Deaconess Hospital, and Harvard, found that the brain's striatum and amygdala begin processing stimuli well before they reach conscious awareness. Keep in mind that the heart talks to these two brain centers via the intrinsic nervous system. Also remember that 65 percent of all sensory awareness is initiated by the heart. Thus, there is dialoguing that takes place from the heart's brain and the "big brain" that reveals a stream of subconscious, sixth-sensory awareness. In other words, the heart's brain processes stimuli first, and then signals to the big brain's neurological reaction centers, which in turn transmit signals to the body.

Our heart, brain, and CNS mechanisms are like a radar defense system that constantly scans our environment for safety. They constantly communicate with one another formulating hypotheses as to what we are likely to soon encounter.

The East has long understood the heart's energetic ability to communicate its wisdom to the rest of the body through the body's energy channels. The ancient Chinese believed the heart to be the home of the mind—the place where quality of life and relationships were governed. They felt that if there was deep unhappiness, the heart would transmit weak ch'i to the rest of the body, forcing the body to have to compensate for the absence of vital life force energy. A joyless heart was seen as one of the chief causal roots of all disease. Like all deficient or excess organs, an unhappy heart is believed to communicate its imbalance to the rest of the body via specific energy channels. A heart imbalance can be energetically diagnosed in many ways, such as a weak pulse on the left wrist, or a visual discoloration on the tip of the tongue. I have found sixth-sensory diagnosis to be one of the more accurate and easy ways to trace heart energy imbalances.

THE SPIRIT OF SIXTH SENSE:
THE ANCIENT EAST

The primary difference between traditional Chinese medicine and classical Chinese medicine is the spiritual and mystical dimension. It has been said that traditional Chinese medicine is an edited form of classical Chinese medicine, intended to meet the more mechanistic standards of the modern world. Classical Chinese medicine, on the other hand, is based on centuries of the intuitive and contemplative insights of sages. It also encompasses theories and practices that draw from literature, astronomy, astrology, and mysticism. It's about so much more than the discipline and technicalities of the body's acupuncture pathways. It's more about attaining a higher wisdom of "the way of things."

Intuition is a topic often written about in ancient and contemporary classical Chinese medical texts. Many theorize that it represents an influence first introduced into the ancient culture by the Huns. In China, intuition is generally thought of as a natural phenomenon and has long been considered an important communication link between the practitioner and the integral body of universal wisdom. It is also believed that the body of universal wisdom can only be accessed through very deep emotional and spiritual concentration. As with Chinese philosophy, classical Chinese medicine ascribes to the philosophy of duality, best characterized by the dualism of yin and yang, and to a belief that balance is of paramount importance. The thought of implementing logic without intuition simply wouldn't occur to them.

Classical Chinese medicine and the spiritual tradition of Taoism are enfolded. *Tao* is often translated as "The Way." Taoist philosophy teaches that it is only by perceiving with the heart that one can come to know the way of truth in all things. When it comes to Chinese Taoist philosophy, intuition is rarely a point of focus.

There is a far greater emphasis placed on the wisdom of an inner knowing, which supersedes both intuition and logic.

Ta Chuech means "To awaken from the dream of life." *Pao-i* translates as "Embrace the one." By awakening from the disintegrated dream of life and embracing integral "oneness," it is believed that we gain access to the flow, unbound by the limitations of the five senses. This doesn't imply entering into any mind states, but rather evolving to a level of realization that results in a greater sixth-sensory awareness.

Ancient Chinese Taoists believed in "a way of things"—a flow and gravity to the nature of life—that pre-exists human manifestation. This is a natural process that, shining through the inherent chaos of the universe, reflects life's order and sequence.

Sixth-sensory awareness is the natural result of mastering the art of "non-doing." By non-doing, I'm referring to clearing the mind of the world's noise to gain access to the silent way of all information. Cultivating and living in such a state of knowing greatly enhanced the diagnostic skills of ancient Chinese medical practitioners. They could anticipate, and therefore prevent, illness and mishaps. They lived and evolved in a state of heightened awareness, allowing for greater sensory access. By evolving their sixth-sensory awareness, they became preeminent physicians. Their innate ability to diagnose and get to the root of physical, emotional, mental, and spiritual imbalances was extraordinary. By grasping and adhering to the way of things, they came to know all things.

OUR MYSTICAL NATURE

Sixth-century philosopher and author of the *Tao Te Ching* Lao Tzu once said: "The power of intuitive understanding will protect you from harm until the end of your days." I have always protected myself, my patients, and all those I love by engaging my sixth-sensory awareness in all that I do. My inclination to bring intuition into my life is merely the result of my deep, abiding compassion. You might say that my mystical nature is a reflection of my spiritual nature. I see it as purely exponential. The more refined your vibration, the more powerful your compassion. If you care about someone, you want to be generous to them. If you care deeply about them, you'll want to give them even more. Inspired by spiritual compassion, I want to give everything I've got. Our spiritual nature seeks to do whatever is necessary to relieve whatever pain and suffering we can. As one of my beloved spiritual teachers, Sri Mata Gyatri Devi, always used to say, "Give it away. Give it all away!"

The word *mystical* is generally defined as having a spiritual reality not apparent to the senses. That's assuming, of course, that our spiritual consciousness doesn't reflect extrasensory awareness. I think of our extrasensory awareness as one innate form of intelligence that we were naturally endowed with. Our mystical nature is a gift that we can choose to develop for our life's greater good, as well as the greater good of those whose lives we touch. I believe that we all have a mystical or spiritual nature that's aligned with higher values, such as compassion, love, and forgiveness. Our human nature emanates from the corporeal self. Our mystical nature emanates from the domains of spirit and soul. These domains represent centers of higher energetic vibration that allow us access to sixth-sensory intelligence.

When our mystical nature is engaged, we're also activating very specific vectors in our brain that operate inductively, or intuitively. If we fail to exercise these areas of our brain, they tend to weaken. If regularly engaged, on the other hand, there's no limit to what we can do with them. It's all about breaking down our resistance to our own mystical nature.

Every culture represents an experiment. Ancient Eastern culture is, for the most part, steeped in a history accented with mysticism.

Our contemporary Western experiment is centered on materialism. It isn't too difficult to figure out why we have decided to exclude sixth-sensory reality altogether. It's neither materially profitable nor is it anything that can be double-blind-control studied. Where our system of medicine is mechanistic, the ancient Chinese system of medicine is vitalistic.

Classical Chinese medicine is based on a system of internal alchemy. This system was all about disciplining its practitioners to sharpen their mystical senses. They believed that nature spoke her own silent language and that only by learning to decipher it could they advance their mystical potential.

Theirs is a message that reminds us that we've all been graced with the innate power to know outcomes well in advance of their onset. They inspire us to tune in deeply within and all around us. For many, sixth-sensory awareness simply doesn't exist. Among an ever-growing population, however, it's believed to hold the secrets of our true mystical nature and its infinite possibilities.

Calming the Five Seas

Many of us are convinced that we have little or no sixth-sensory awareness. Nothing could be further from the truth. Calming the Five Seas and Merging with the Great Sea are two very powerful Whole Health exercises designed to strengthen your command of your sixth-sensory awareness. Classical Chinese medicine teaches that we have three vital energy centers, or "seas of ch'i," called *dantiens*. These seas of energy are responsible for the storage and cultivation of our life energy. There is a lower, middle, and upper sea. Along with these three vital energy points, Whole Health includes two vital points in its Calming the Five Seas energy protocol. The addition of these two acupuncture points (CV 12 and CV 22) will better enable you to clear your mind of clutter and anxiety, opening you up to a clearer stream of consciousness.

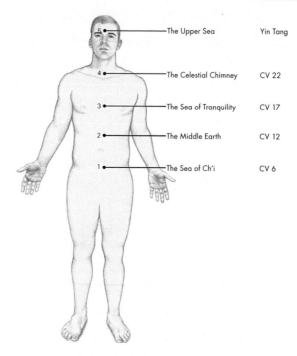

The Upper Sea	Yin Tang	
The Celestial Chimney	CV 22	
The Sea of Tranquility	CV 17	
The Middle Earth	CV 12	
The Sea of Ch'i	CV 6	

FIGURE 3.1   *Balancing the Five Seas*

1. The first acupuncture point is the lower sea, also called the Sea of Ch'i, and is located approximately two fingers below the navel and two fingers behind the skin. It is Conception Vessel 6, or CV 6 (see Figure 3.1). The lower sea corresponds with the kidneys and controls thoughts and feelings. The lower sea is thought to be the energy center responsible for grounding, or rooting. This is where one can settle down one's nervous system from the destabilizing influences of negative thoughts and restless emotions.

2. The second point is called the Middle Earth. It is located between the first and second seas, four fingers above the navel and two fingers behind the skin. This is the Conception Vessel 12 acupuncture point, or CV 12, noted for calming obsessive thinking.

3. The third point, or middle sea, is often called the Sea of Tranquility. The middle sea is located two fingers behind the heart. This is the Conception Vessel 17 acupuncture point, or CV 17. This point corresponds with both the emotional and physical heart, as well as the thymus gland. It is associated with emotion, immunity, vitality, and the overall health of the internal glands and organs.

4. The fourth point is called the Celestial Chimney, located between the second and third seas, in the center of the suprasternal fossa. It is Conception Vessel 22, or CV 22. Among other things, this point is noted for calming rising anxiety and stress.

5. The fifth and final point is the upper sea, located at the forehead, between the eyes, and two fingers behind the center point between the eyebrows. Often called the Central Mark, the upper sea corresponds with the pineal gland and is responsible for governance over the higher consciousness, intellect, and wisdom of the spirit.

Once in balance, we are then able to expand our energy field so as to be able to merge our personal seas of energy with the great universal sea of energy. The whole purpose of Merging with the Great Sea is to attain greater powers of sixth-sensory energy diagnosis and healing. I was spiritually guided to develop this exercise a number of years ago. It continues to successfully assist many sixth-sensory practitioners of energy medicine.

The exercise is simple and should be practiced often and just before engaging in EMT diagnostic testing (see chapter 4). If practiced properly, Merging with the Great Sea will transform one's sixth-sensory adeptness in no time and with little effort.

Before beginning this exercise, it is important to prepare properly. Make sure you are comfortable and in a quiet environment with little or no distraction. Turn off all phones, and put the Do Not Disturb sign on the door. This entire exercise shouldn't take more than fifteen minutes, but it requires quiet concentration.

Clearing the Mortal Haze is initiated by taking three deep breaths. Begin by breathing out until you can't empty your lungs any more. Hold the exhale for three full seconds. Then slowly take your first full inhale until you can't fill your lungs with any more air. Hold the breath in for a full three seconds. Now, while still holding the breath, open your mouth, count to three, and exhale with your mouth wide open. Make sure to once again fully clear the lungs. Now slowly take your second full inhale, making sure to fill your lungs fully again, and hold the breath for a count of three. Again, open your mouth while still holding your breath, and count to three. Exhale with your mouth fully open and completely clear your lungs of the breath. Now take your third and final inhale, making sure to really fill your lungs. Hold the breath in for a full three seconds. Again, hold the breath in, open your mouth, and continue to hold for a full count of three. With mouth fully open, release your third and final clearing exhale. Now you are ready to begin Merging with the Great Sea.

You may practice this exercise either sitting or standing. Remember, without being too concerned about keeping exact time, each of the five Merging exercises should last for approximately three minutes.

Now, as you begin, remain relaxed, with eyes closed.

Merging with the Great Sea

1. *Clearing the Mortal Haze*—This balances the first sea of ch'i and clears fear, anxiety, and confusion. As with each of the following exercises, one should begin Clearing the Mortal Haze fully relaxed and seated with eyes closed. Next, place both hands (left under right for men and right under left for women) over your navel and focus all of your mind's attention there. Envision healing radiant sunlight traveling down both of your arms and depositing into your lower *dantien*. As the light travels down your

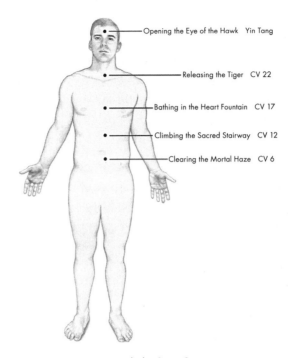

Opening the Eye of the Hawk   Yin Tang

Releasing the Tiger   CV 22

Bathing in the Heart Fountain   CV 17

Climbing the Sacred Stairway   CV 12

Clearing the Mortal Haze   CV 6

FIGURE 3.2   *Merging with the Great Sea*

arms and hands, at last arriving at your *dantien*, picture it spinning in a counterclockwise spiral direction (you are the clock, facing outward—this means your incoming energy spiral will be spinning to your right). This is an important Wenchiech'u technique that will markedly increase the incoming ch'i. (The following chapters will discuss Wenchiech'u in greater detail.) This exercise should last no more than three minutes.

The keyword for this exercise is *clear*. Clearing the Mortal Haze is designed to shut down your brain's production of beta brain waves (stress brain waves), shifting it over to an alpha brain wave state (relaxation). This will assist you in transforming your mortal mind.

2. *Climbing the Sacred Stairway*—This balances the second sea and clears obsessive tendencies. Begin by placing both hands over

the area between your navel and your heart. Once again, focus all your attention there and once again envision streams of sunlight running down your arms and hands to fill up this area of your attention. Don't forget to spin the sunlight energy counterclockwise. The keyword for this exercise is *elevate*. Climbing the Sacred Stairway is designed to align your body and mind with your intention to begin elevating your energy to the highest possible vibration. Remember, your intention is to elevate your energy so as to open up your mystical self. This will enable you to gain access to your highest sixth-sensory potential.

3. *Bathing in the Heart Fountain*—This exercise balances the third sea and clears emotional distortions. To begin Bathing in the Heart Fountain, place both hands over your heart, and as you do, visualize healing sunlight energy moving down both arms and hands, filling up your heart. Once again, spin the energy counterclockwise. The keyword for this exercise is *compassion*. As you fill up your heart center with healing energy, feel that energy beginning to generate a fountainhead and imagine yourself bathing in a radiant light of love. It is very important here to focus your intention on attaining your deepest level of compassion. Compassion in service is the most vivifying energy that inspires and potentiates our sixth-sensory potential.

4. *Releasing the Tiger*—This balances the fourth sea of ch'i. Releasing the Tiger requires that you place both hands over the area just beneath your throat. This will open up the mystical voice of the spirit and enable one to express their higher truth. Again visualize healing sunlight being drawn down the arms and hands into that area. Now spin the sunlight in counterclockwise spirals. The keyword for this exercise is *will*. One must strive to merge their compassion with gamma brain waves at this point. Gamma brain waves may be thought of as waves generated by great undisturbed focus and powerful intention. So, when Re-

leasing the Tiger, one empowers their compassion with a focus and a determined intention.

5. *Opening the Eyes of the Hawk*—This balances the fifth sea and opens up the stream of higher consciousness. The keyword for this exercise is *transcend*. Place both hands over the area between your eyebrows, and once again picture streams of healing energy flowing into that area. Next, spin the energy counterclockwise and, as you do this, remember that this exercise represents the final step of your effort to elevate your body, mind, and spirit energies to a place far beyond your everyday self.

For those developing sixth-sensory consciousness, these developmental exercises should be practiced routinely. Once your sixth sense is better developed, you'll be ready to master assessing, balancing, and preserving your mutable constitution through Whole Health Energy Diagnosis.

CHAPTER 4

WHOLE HEALTH ENERGY DIAGNOSIS

THE SYSTEM'S ROOTS

In chapter 2, I discussed how to establish your fixed constitution. Chapter 3 helped you connect with your sixth-sense self. Now you are ready to begin learning how to diagnose and balance your mutable constitution. There are a myriad of changing energies that continuously affect our vital glands and organs each day. Climate, weather, diet, relationships, and other shifting events are all representative of catalysts for change. The fluidity of life is forever bringing its influences to bear on our vital glands and organs, and thus our overall health. This variability is particularly challenging to anyone espousing a lifestyle of disease prevention.

Whole Health Body Energy Diagnosis is an electromagnetic muscle-testing system specifically designed to monitor the body's energy fluctuations. Before detailing this further, I must first familiarize you with some basic fundamentals of classical Chinese medicine. In the following Yin-Yang list, the first organ is governed by yin, the second by yang.

The Five Elements Organ System

Yin-Yang

1. Liver–gallbladder
2. Heart–small intestine
3. Spleen–stomach
4. Lung–large intestine
5. Kidney–bladder

The ancient Chinese embraced the philosophy of "mutual compatibility of opposites." This was the first constitutional distinction made between all things. Everything between heaven and earth was seen as having either a yin or a yang nature. Yin is a metaphor for the female principle: passive, dark, cold, inner, winter, descending, hollow, and so on. Yang represents the male principle: active, light, hot, summer, ascending, solid, and so on. Thus, the vital organs are classified as either yin or yang.

It is very important to keep in mind that yin and yang are not static states. Yin and yang are fluid, dynamic states that are forever flowing into each other. Yin may be the opposite of yang, but it is always in the active process of becoming yang, and vice versa. Every great fire burns intensely (yang), but is destined to swiftly burn itself out (yin). Even the hardest monsoon rains (yin) are in the process of eventually giving way to the hot tropical sun (yang). Even the newborn baby (yang) is aging, and thus part of the slow, gradual process of surrendering its material existence (yin). This dichotomy is true for organ system relationships as well. Each yin organ, such as the liver, performs yang tasks, such as managing the body's energy. By the same token, each yang organ, like the gall-bladder, has an important yin influence, such as the secretion of bile, which is extremely alkaline (yin). Our task is to manage the balance between our yin and yang influences.

These organ systems represent human energy conduits that determine and reflect one's degree of wellness-balance, or *harmony.* Any energy imbalances in these organ systems represent a *disharmony.* For example, to communicate harshly with a patient, using verbiage that generates dis-ease, may result in negative mental and emotional energy that further damages their spirit and lessens their prospect for recovery. All patterns of dis-ease are the result of imbalances and referred to as *disharmonies.*

One of the most important diagnostic points is to establish whether a patient's organ disharmonies are internally or externally rooted.

1. *External disharmony*—physical, cellular, material origin (yang)
2. *Internal disharmony*—mental, emotional, spiritual origin (yin)

Before any effective treatment protocol can be established, both practitioner and patient must know where the energy disharmony is rooted. External disharmonies will require greater cellular support like nutrition. Internal disharmonies will require more energetic support, like homeopathy, Qigong, or T'ai Chi.

Once again, practitioners should be reminded that when it comes to energy diagnosis, there are only three possible energies:

1. Excess (disharmony)
2. Deficiency (disharmony)
3. Balance (harmony)

When the energy of an organ is diagnosed as *excess,* it suggests that there is too much energy in that organ. This may be thought of as *inflammatory.* When an organ is *deficient,* it means there is not enough energy in that organ. This may be thought of as *degenerative.*

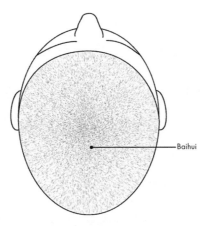

FIGURE 4.1   *Baihui*

The goal of this energy work is to *balance* all the vital organ airs and bring the subject to optimal health. Before we actually go on to describe the diagnostic evaluation, there are three fundamental questions that we need to look at:

1. "Where does ch'i come from?"

Powerful yang ch'i descends into the body from the heavens and enters the body through Governing Vessel 20 (GV 20). This point, located dead center on top of the head and directly up from both ears, is also called *Baihui* (See Figure 4.1). In the Chinese tradition, *Baihui* is where our highest spiritual energies converge. This point correlates with the Thousand Petal Lotus, or Sacred Crown Chakra, common to Eastern Indian thought. Many other religions and spiritual traditions have depicted the sacred energy of this crown region with an aura, or halo. *Baihui* marks the yang ch'i entry point.

Conception Vessel 1 (CV 1), or *Hui-Yin* point (located in the perineum between the genitals and the anus), is where the earthly yin energies enter the body. It is also referred to as the meeting place of yin.

Baihui delivers the flow of heavenly yang ch'i down the back of the body, and *Hui-Yin* draws the flow of turbid, earthly energy up the front of the body. This two-way flow between the gates of life and death creates what is called the Microcosmic Orbit. Only when the two gates are vivified and balanced can there be abundant life force. To both regulate and balance these vital gates, one need only meditate on the Microcosmic Orbit of their own ch'i. Relaxed and with eyes closed, take a breath and visualize the radiant flow of these respective energies. Continue to envision the orbiting energy cycling down the back and up the front of your body for five to seven minutes. Perform this exercise as often as possible. This is a foundational and powerful meditation technique to have in your repertoire.

The heavens are considered the source of cosmic and prenatal energy. Cosmic energy in the form of light is believed to enter into the body through the top of the head, eyes, and skin. Prenatal essence (like DNA) is passed on from the parents into the womb. There is also a cosmic prenatal force believed to be carried over from past lives. Therefore, we are told that when a child is born, he or she brings a certain degree of life-force energy from previous incarnations.

Ch'i also ascends up into the body from the earth, in the form of energies transferred to us from the earth's food, water, and herbs. Ch'i is also provided by the human processes of respiration (oxygen), digestion (food), circulation (blood), and detoxification. Oxygen and food are at the top of the life-force energy list. Keep in mind that 75 percent of the human body is water, and 90 percent of water is oxygen. When food is digested, it is distilled by the spleen and then transformed into blood.

2. "How does excess ch'i come to accumulate in an organ?"

First, there is the issue of fixed, prenatal constitution. Someone may simply be born with a tendency to specific imbalances. It is also important to keep in mind that excess energy may be the result of a blockage that builds up from mutable, postnatal constitutional influences, such as lifestyle or diet. For example, too much fatty food in the diet may be obstructing the movement of bile in the liver, creating an external hepatic excess. Another example might be if someone is repressing sadness—this can create an internal disharmony in the lung, or generate an excess of pulmonary energy.

3. "How does deficient ch'i come to manifest in an organ?"

Again we must consider pre- and postnatal constitution influences. We must also remember that day-to-day influences like an excess of stress (internal disharmony), insufficient sleep, or inadequate nutrition can create deficiencies in virtually all organs.

THE EXTERNAL CAUSES OF DISEASE

When it comes to fully understanding the rooting of disharmony/ ch'i imbalances, the most important considerations are the Six Pernicious Influences, the Five Flavors, and the Five Emotions. These influences represent those common energies most inclined to imbalance vital organ systems.

The Six Pernicious Influences

1. *Wind*—Injures the liver—Protect yourself from strong wind, sudden changes, and impulsive angers.
2. *Heat* (mild heat)—Injures the heart—Eat cool foods in summer and remain relaxed at all times.
3. *Fire* (severe heat)—Injures the heart—Don't overexert the body in summer, and avoid emotional mania and intense frustration.
4. *Dampness*—Injures the spleen—Eat dry food when the weather is damp, and warm yourself with your own compassion.
5. *Dryness*—Injures the lungs—Hydrate when it's dry and balance your release of tears.
6. *Cold*—Injures the kidneys—Dress warmly, eat warm foods in

the cold, and don't let your fear deep-freeze you! (See the Five Emotions, below.)

The Five Flavors

1. *Sour* (for example, lemons)—Imbalances may cause external liver–gallbladder disharmony.
2. *Bitter* (for example, escarole greens)—Imbalances may cause disharmony in the external heart–small intestine.
3. *Sweet* (for example, bananas)—Imbalances may cause external spleen–stomach disharmony.
4. *Pungent* (for example, onions)—Imbalances may cause external lung–large intestine disharmony.
5. *Salty* (for example, celery)—Imbalances may cause external kidney–bladder disharmony.

The Five Emotions

1. *Anger*—Imbalances may cause internal liver–gallbladder disharmony.
2. *Joy*—Imbalances may cause internal heart–small intestine disharmony.
3. *Anxiety*—Imbalances may cause internal spleen–stomach disharmony.
4. *Grief*—Imbalances may cause internal lung–large intestine disharmony.
5. *Fear*—Imbalances may cause internal kidney–bladder disharmony.

ASSESS, BALANCE, AND PRESERVE CH'I

The primary goal of the Whole Health Healing System is to assess, balance, and preserve ch'i through energy diagnostics, diet, lifestyle, mind management, and Qigong (energy exercises). When the vital organs are energetically imbalanced in any way, everything will be out of balance.

Our vital organs are like energy generators that transmit and receive ch'i reciprocally to and from our cells, blood, tissues, emotions, thoughts, spirits, and souls (mortal and immortal). Each of us is an interconnected microuniverse of energy that is regulated by and through our vital organs. Each organ system is like a separate galaxy in charge of regulating the gravitational movements of its star systems and, in so doing, it contributes to the wholeness of a universe of energy. For example, if our diet contains an overabundance of fat, the liver–gallbladder can suffer from an excess of ch'i, which can then trigger extreme fits of anger and exhaust our nervous system. If we fail to balance our excess worry, our spleen–stomach will tend to generate an uncontrollable desire for sugar, and our digestive tract will become inflamed. Energetically speaking, every aspect of our total being is interrelated, interdependent, and overseen by our vital organs. The heart is not only in charge of our circulation; it also works closely with the small intestines, and manages our mental willpower. Besides regulating our respiration, the lungs also help us to maintain moisture in the large intestine, enhance our intuition, and enable us to overcome our grief.

In order to attain wholeness, the energies that flow within and from our vital organ systems demand that ch'i be constantly assessed, balanced, and preserved.

THE CH'I BODY CLOCK

The Ch'i Body Clock assessment is one of the simplest ways to tap into vital organ disharmonies (see Figure 4.2). The ancient Chinese believed that ch'i entered into the organ systems at specific times and that by being aware of the state of our body energy during those times, we could learn a great deal about our organ system

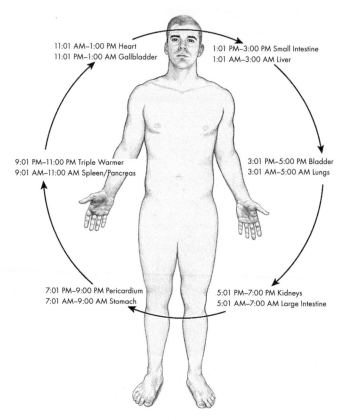

11:01 AM–1:00 PM Heart
11:01 PM–1:00 AM Gallbladder

1:01 PM–3:00 PM Small Intestine
1:01 AM–3:00 AM Liver

9:01 PM–11:00 PM Triple Warmer
9:01 AM–11:00 AM Spleen/Pancreas

3:01 PM–5:00 PM Bladder
3:01 AM–5:00 AM Lungs

7:01 PM–9:00 PM Pericardium
7:01 AM–9:00 AM Stomach

5:01 PM–7:00 PM Kidneys
5:01 AM–7:00 AM Large Intestine

FIGURE 4.2   *The Ch'i Body Clock*

balances and imbalances. For example, if someone is frequently awakened and their sleep disturbed between 1:00 a.m. and 3:00 a.m., it would indicate excess liver ch'i. If someone experiences extreme fatigue each evening between 5:00 p.m. and 7:00 p.m., it would indicate deficient kidney ch'i. It is important to include these body clock assessments as part of a greater global awareness of self. For example, if one is grieving the loss of a loved one, is experiencing labored breathing (lungs), and is awakening frequently between 3:00 a.m. and 5:00 a.m. they would likely be suffering from lung ch'i deficiency. Grief, lung debilitation, and restlessness between 3:00 a.m. and 5:00 a.m. are all lung markers.

MUSCLE TESTING

Whole Health has developed its own customized system of neuro-muscular biofeedback as a vehicle for assessing, balancing, and pre-serving ch'i. Classical Chinese medicine represents a 5,000-year-old history of human energy diagnostics. I credit those ancient masters as the true originators and progenitors of muscle testing. Applied kinesiology (muscle testing) as we know it today was formally founded by Dr. George Goodheart in the early 1960s. A quick definition of applied kinesiology (AK) is that it is a muscle-testing biofeedback procedure that allows a practitioner quick, easy access to discovering energetic body imbalances between cells, nerves, muscles, and organ systems.

Goodheart discovered that each large muscle in the body energetically correlates to specific major gland and organ systems, which are tied together by nerve cells. This connection (neuromus-cular) between nerve and muscle is what makes the muscles so reactive and so revealing of conditions in the body and mind. Goodheart's remarkable muscle testing system incorporated ele-ments of his genius as a chiropractor.

Over the past several decades, many additional contributions have been made to the art and science of muscle testing. Dr. John Diamond developed a system of muscle testing he called behavioral kinesiology. This was also a biofeedback form of muscle testing, but it focused more on the influences the mind has over the body's cells, nerves, muscles, and organs. Where Goodheart's approach was based on the physical, Diamond's was more psychological. In the years that followed, other pioneers, such as Drs. John Thie, David Leaf, John Campbell, Richard Versendaal, and David Haw-kins, were among the many that made noteworthy contributions to understanding this great diagnostic tool.

Today there are a number of muscle-testing systems, each with its own unique approaches and theories. This one-of-a-kind healing art serves as a testament to the great traditions in energy diagnostics, such as classical Chinese medicine. Like classical Chinese medicine, muscle testing has been free to evolve without the restriction of standardization or regulation. For the most part, there have been no oppressive governing bodies or administrative structures set in place to stunt its growth. It's always been about healing masters that have passed down their insights from generation to generation. Each practitioner remains free to add their own unique insights to an ever-evolving, healing art form. Any natural phenomenon such as human neuromuscular biofeedback should serve as a reminder that the ways of nature are not invented—they are merely discovered and shared.

WHOLE HEALTH ELECTROMAGNETIC MUSCLE TESTING (EMT)

EMT allows practitioner and subject to diagnostically assess and regulate mutable constitutionality in a dynamic, natural way. Nature has designed our defense system to be one of our most powerful and consistently reliable mechanisms. This is because nature's greatest priority is for the survival of our species. Thus, as was discussed in chapter 3, we've been given sixth-sensory awareness. As such, our protective alarm systems have been designed with an extrasensory hair trigger intended to respond to virtually all perceived stimuli, even if only imagined. As we saw earlier, when you intuitively anticipate a negative outcome or have a bad dream, your heart rate will elevate. Intuitive thoughts and dreams alone are more than enough to set off our defense system's neurological triggers. Our bodies, minds, and spirits remain at the ready to respond to any and all stimuli. Such is the way of our protective sixth-sensory biofeedback. This response is first registered by our nerves and muscles—the neuromuscular system. To interpret the messages from our neuromuscular biofeedback system, one can simply try an exercise I introduced you to earlier, where a subject lifts their arm and attempts to resist as a practitioner depresses their arm while presenting a variety of verbal stimuli. Words alone produce images in the mind that are more than capable of activating or de-activating the nerves within our muscles. And, as with the dream example, it doesn't take much to activate our alarm systems. Words alone will trigger a positive or negative biofeedback response. For example, a word like *danger* will generally be more than enough to weaken one's neuromuscular biofeedback response, while the word *happiness* will tend to strengthen it.

There are twelve applications that make up the Whole Health EMT system. These twelve are comprised of four basic, four primary, and two secondary applications, as well as two self-testing techniques. There is also a supplemental longevity application offered at the end of this chapter. In order for students to properly learn this energy system, they must first master each of the twelve applications in proper sequence.

The Four Basic EMT Applications

1. *EMT Pass/Fail Position and Testing*—Before you begin testing, the practitioner will need to obtain a sugar packet such as is used to sweeten coffee. Next, the practitioner and subject stand face-to-face at arm's-length distance (see Figure 4.3). Practitioners should employ their dominant hand as their test hand because the dominant hand is more sensitive to energetic subtleties. (But, as the practitioner becomes more experienced, they should alternate hands so as not to become right/left imbalanced.) Next, the practitioner should instruct the subject to raise their left arm (provided the practitioner is right dominant), slightly higher than shoulder height. Then, ask them to clench the fist of their raised (test) hand. Next, instruct the subject to resist as you gently attempt to depress their raised and arm wrist with your dominant hand as you push evenly and lightly on the subject's wrist. Just

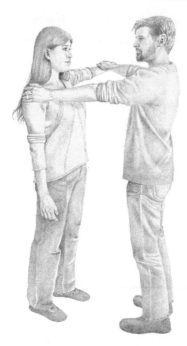

FIGURE 4.3   EMT Pass/Fail Position

spend the next three to five minutes getting accustomed to the strength and resistance tendencies of your subject. Remember, you are partners who are very much reliant on each other for accurate results. So take some time to establish a good energy rapport with each other. Soon you should have a pretty good idea what your subject's test strength baseline feels like. The test strength baseline is the same as a test pass strength. Once test pass strength is determined, it should be easy to distinguish a test fail. With your free hand, hold a sugar packet close to the subject's heart and give their test arm a light tug at the wrist. This is a most assured way to guarantee a fail test result.

2. *EMT Tuning*—Tuning will take you to the next level beyond pass/fail. Once again, practitioner and subject must assume pass/fail position. To bring practitioner and subject better in tune with each other, the practitioner should begin by simply

calling out a negative word such as *hopelessness*, while simultaneously administering a pass/fail muscle test. Just from hearing
a negative word, the subject will record the energy of the
word at a neuromuscular level, prompting a failed muscle test. If
need be, practitioners should make several attempts to get a
fail response. You might even consider trying other negative
words. One negative word may have a more powerful influence
on a given subject than another. Clearly, some negative word—
hopelessness, cancer, or *lonely*—will produce a natural loss in the
subject's arm strength. Now, repeat the exact same tuning procedure, but this time call out a positive word like *vibrant*. Again,
repeat it several times, until you establish a strong, resistant,
positive arm response. You might try other positive words, such
as *happy, healthy,* or *love,* just to establish clear tuning. Tuning is
absolutely essential in order to establish a good testing rapport
between practitioner and subject. Remember, EMT is an extrasensory muscle-testing system. The sources of biofeedback information are the practitioner's and subject's intuitions, generated
by the cardiac intrinsic ganglia and transmitted to mind, brain,
and body.

3. *EMT Pulse Testing*—Pulse testing enables the Whole Health
practitioner and subject to determine the exact relative score of
any given muscle test. With tuning, you were able to discover
the sharp contrasts in muscle strength between positive and negative words. With pulse testing, you will determine the exact degree of positive and negative influence virtually any influences
(words, foods, vitamins) have on your subject. In order to begin
pulse testing, the practitioner and subject must first assume pass/
fail positioning. Now let's assume the subject failed a tuning test
when hearing the practitioner call out the word *hopeless*. The
practitioner must first announce aloud that they are going to test
exactly how negatively the word *hopeless* affects the subject's nervous system in relative numbers between minus 1 and minus 10,

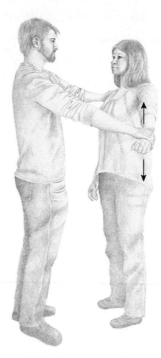

FIGURE 4.4   *Pulse Testing*

with minus 10 representing the most negative effect. Then the practitioner will call out the word *hopeless* once again and instead of just pushing down the subject's arm, this time the practitioner will try pulsing their arm while slowly counting from minus 1 to minus 10 (see Figure 4.4). If their arm drops at minus 1, the word isn't having a severely negative effect. If the subject's test arm remains strong until a count of minus 10, however, it indicates that the word is having an extremely negative effect on their neuromuscular system, etc. The same pulse testing can be performed for positive responses from plus 1 to plus 10 as well. Pulse testing can also be utilized for organ testing, food testing, and focus reliability testing. More about that in a moment.

4. *EMT Focus/Reliability*—Focus/Reliability is a procedure that technically might best be performed before any other EMT protocols, but by advanced students only! Beginners must first es-

tablish familiarity with pass/fail position testing, tuning, and pulse testing. Focus reliability enables practitioner and subject to ensure that they are both integrally focused, intentionally clear, and energetically accurate. When pulse testing for focus/reliability, the practitioner should first verbally pose the following question to the subject: "What is our present degree of focus/reliability from one to ten, with ten being the highest number?" Then you should attempt to gently pulse test the subject's arm at the wrist with a "one at a time" push approach, while counting out from one to ten as they do. When the subject's arm weakens and drops, you'll have arrived at your focus/reliability factor. Note that nothing less than 10 is acceptable! If the score is lower, simply ask that both of you consciously acknowledge your lack of focus/reliability, and then immediately remedy the problem with a higher commitment and mental focus from both of you. In other words, you must establish accuracy before performing any further testing! I've found that by merely calling attention to the lack of focus/reliability, things usually snap right in place. Once again, the practitioner pushes down on their partner's arm and calls out score numbers from 1 to 10. This is typically all it takes to get the focus/reliability up to 10. Now that you have completed the five preliminary EMT protocols, you are ready to commence with the principal EMT vital organ, organ root reference, and food testing protocols.

The Four Primary EMT Applications

1. *EMT Vital Organ Testing* (Long Form Chart) represents the first of the primary Whole Health energy assessment techniques. This procedure enables the practitioner to diagnose a subject's body, brain, mind, emotions, and spirit energies. In order to get started, practitioners will need the three-page EMT Long Form (Appendix B). The first part is designed for body, the second part for brain, and the third part for mind assessment.

The upper half of page one lists the five pairs of vital organs. The vital organs listed here represent the Five Elements organ systems of classical Chinese medicine. The lower half lists the primary glands. These worksheets were specifically designed to enable the Whole Health practitioner to record the subject's energy responses. Let's get started.

Practitioners must begin by pass/fail testing the subject's vital organs in sequence as they appear on the EMT chart. The liver should be tested first, followed by gallbladder, heart, small intestine, and so on. Practitioners must follow the pass/fail testing technique for the vital organs and glands. It is a simple procedure. Practitioners simply apply light pressure with the left hand to the subject's organ zone being tested. Advanced practitioners can either just call out, or merely think about the organ area being tested as they pulse the strength of the subject's test arm with their dominant hand. The light pulsing of the subject's arm strength as the corresponding organ zones are being depressed should proceed through a count of ten. In other words, if pressure is applied to the organ point and the test arm is weak or strong, you'll need to pulse exactly how weak or strong it is, plus/minus 1 to 10.

If the test arm weakens and drops after a count of one, two, three, or four tugs, then the organ should be considered to be only slightly energized. If the test arm weakens and drops at a pulse count of four, five, or six, then it is only moderately strong. If the arm drops after seven, eight, or nine pulses, organ energy is sufficiently strong. If it pulses to a count of ten, it is perfectly balanced. Excess organ strength (inflammation) is measured by pulse counts that exceed ten, to a count of twenty or higher. EMT vital organ testing requires both a complete pass/fail and a pulse test assessment, which must be checked, double-checked, and properly recorded on the EMT Long Form Chart (see Appendix B).

2. *Root Reference Testing*—Next, the organ root reference must be established. This assists the practitioner in finding out whether the root cause of the organ/gland imbalance is due to diet, mental, emotional, chemical, or structural problems. Remember, this is not a system that ascribes to treating symptoms. Whole Health emphasizes the importance of tracing back to the roots of all disease patterns. This enables a practitioner to more effectively and safely treat the subject. Treating the symptoms and not the root is one of the main reasons for serious medical side effects.

A dietary root, of course, suggests that whatever the subject's symptoms are, they are best addressed at the nutritional level. Mental roots represent more of a stress-related patterning. Where organ imbalances are found, there may need to be recommendations for neuroplasticity exercises, meditation, yoga, T'ai Chi, Bach flower remedies, or classic homeopathy. An emotional root also tends to represent stress-related patterning, and issues related to the spirit. The Shen Clearing exercise in chapter 8 may be necessary for the subject to clear out old emotional blockages that are deeply rooted sources of energy imbalances. If a chemical root is established, it represents exposures to toxic substances such as pesticides, mercury amalgams, drugs, household chemicals, and so on. This diagnostic discovery may require some form of detoxification or chelation. Finally, structural imbalance resulting from past physical traumas, accidents, or sports injuries are also common roots practitioners may discover.

At the bottom of page 303 additional diagnostic markers for bacteria, staph, mold, strep, cranial yeast, sacral yeast, infectious virus, retrovirus, and a gland/organ root reference. Each of these markers should also be pass/fail and pulse tested to give the practitioner a greater depth of immunological information about the subject.

The second part (EMT Brain Assessment) is broken down

into four brain systems: cerebral cortex, limbic system, cerebellum, and brain stem. Each of these sections is briefly defined so as to provide both practitioner and subject with some referencing for their energy testing. Once again, if a failed muscle test is recorded, the corresponding brain assessment should be crossed out. Next, a pulse test will either be noted with a specific minus/plus 1–10 score, which may be entered on the corresponding blank space to the right-hand side of the page.

Finally, the chart presents practitioner and subject with a Mind Assessment part. There are four state of mind categories listed here: conscious (alert), unconscious (trance), metaconscious (higher), and superconscious (highest) mind. The same exact test procedures are to be followed for mind as for body and brain assessment—pass/fail and pulse testing, with plus/minus 1–10 scores recorded in the blank spaces on the right.

3. *Food Vial Allergy Testing*—The Food Vial Allergy Testing technique employs homeopathic food testing vials. Actual foods may be used for food muscle testing, but the homeopathic vials are much more convenient and efficient. This simple pass/fail approach to food allergy testing represents the very first muscle testing procedure I performed decades ago. In fact, I first started with real whole foods. There was a supermarket directly across the street from the medical center where I worked. So when patients called to schedule their initial work-ups, I suggested they purchase their groceries across the street just prior to our meeting. That way, I could muscle test them for exactly those foods they were most accustomed to eating. Then I was introduced to homeopathic food vials. They were initially used for Vega machine testing, a mechanical system whereby patients could be electronically tested while holding drops from the foods vials under the tongue. I remember thinking how silly that was. People were largely unaware back then as to the ways of energy and energy fields. I was pretty clear, due to my energy

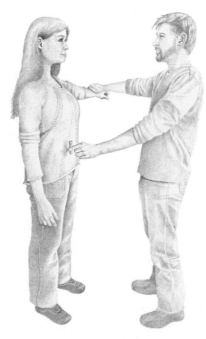

FIGURE 4.5   *Vial Testing*

awareness, about the fact that the homeopathic food vials produced a very active field and would need only to be held close
to the subject to elicit a viable pass/fail energy result. The vials
I recommend are made by Apex Energetics in Irvine, California.
These little glass vials (kits 1 and 2) contain homeopathic dilutions of hundreds of common foods, and these diluted foods
emit a field of highly active energy. In fact, the more diluted
their material properties, the more powerful their energy. I can
hear your thoughts as you read this. "The more diluted the material properties in these vials, the more powerful their energy?"
Just try thinking of the relationship between energy and matter
as creating a drawstring-like effect. As matter is diminished, energy increases, and vice versa. Moreover, we must remember
that energy is not bound by material restriction. Sound waves in
the next room are audible right through the wall. Similarly, the

field emitted from the food vials projects outside the glass when held next to the field of a human being. You will get a reaction! Let's move on with the testing.

Assuming you and your partner are back in test position, you merely have to repeat the tuning procedure. Then grab a food vial and hold it close to your partner (see Figure 4.5). I suggest you hold the food vials next to wherever the patient's "pain point" is. For instance, if the patient has a history of headaches, ask them to point out exactly where their headaches tend to occur. That is what I call their "pain point." Depending on the subject, their pain point may be their stomach, an inflamed shoulder, or whatever else is ailing them.

As with tuning, the food vial exposures will produce both positive and negative strength results. When a problem food is held close to your partner's arm, the arm will weaken and easily drop to their side with a light tug. Before beginning actual pass/fail vial testing, make sure you ask your partner to check off a food list of only those foods they eat and enjoy the most. There is no point in testing them for foods they don't eat or like. Take your time and test as many foods as they are willing to. Make sure you date and record your results.

4. *EMT Food Allergy Testing*—Now that you've assessed body, mind, and spirit balance and performed food vial allergy testing, it's time for EMT food and supplement testing. Unlike food vial allergy testing, EMT food allergy testing is a sixth-sensory body/mind technique. I always remind people that your energy field will respond to the energy field of whole foods, homeopathic foods in vials, or even just the mention of foods. Remember, your body/mind responds to virtually all stimuli, so don't be afraid to get very specific when articulating your questions. The body/mind will also respond to any questions regarding amount, dose, frequency, and duration. Make sure you have your EMT Food Chart nearby (Appendix C). Now, assuming you and your

subject are in proper position, the tester simply calls out each food in sequence, one at a time, and tries to depress the subject's arm as each food is called out. If the arm goes down while calling out a certain food, you should cross it off the food list. That food should be avoided until it is retested in four to six weeks.

I am often asked how it's possible to be tested for food allergies without physical exposure to foods. Perhaps a little more information might prove helpful. As discussed in earlier chapters, EMT is an energy diagnostic system. In order to fully appreciate EMT as a food-testing medium, we must consider some fundamental properties of energy. As previously discussed, all things, including you and me, are comprised of energy. All energy is made up of atoms and particles. Atoms and particles vibrate, producing an electromagnetic field. Therefore you and I, the thoughts we think (intuitive and logical), and the foods we eat all produce a vibrating electromagnetic (energetic) field. Humans emit 0.025 volts of electricity and 100 watts of radiation in the infrared spectrum. Therefore, we constantly emit ever-changing energy that influences and is influenced by all other energies. Your energy changes when you don't sleep, hug a friend, write a check, catch the flu, dream a dream, think a thought, or eat a food. Furthermore, every dream, friend, virus, or food emits its own unique field of ever-changing energy. So, in the energy domain, fields are constantly interacting with and influencing one other, ad infinitum. While you may not be immediately aware of it, your energy field reacts positively or negatively whenever you eat a food. Your energy field reacts even when a food is in your hand, near your body, or in your mind! By simply closing your eyes and picturing a food in your mind, you will produce a reaction in your energy field. Like all energetic reactions, it will be either a positive or a negative reaction. The reaction may be too subtle for you to notice on the spot, but it is a reaction that greatly influences your degree of overall wellness. EMT allows us to pinpoint positive and negative food reactions at an energetic level, with the unconscious mind. Let's walk you through a test.

First, you and your partner must assume the proper position. Then simply call out the names of foods one at a time as you gently tug on your partner's wrist. Take the time to carefully assess the reaction to each separate food. Remember, simply calling out the words *apple, broccoli,* or *wheat* produces an energetic response in you and your partner. It's merely a different form of tuning test. It's a simple procedure, but keep in mind there's a lot going on here. Your thoughts about the food mentioned emit an electromagnetic field. After all, thoughts are things! Both you and your partner produce an electromagnetic response to any given stimulus in your intuitive unconscious mind that passes to the brain, the nervous system, and the muscles. Both you and your partner have in essence become active biofeedback systems. With a good rapport, you should be able to test dozens of food responses in a matter of mere minutes.

Another very important practice is the act of classifying food reactions. Whole Health subscribes to what it calls Traffic Light Classification. That is, over time, every food will ultimately fall into one of three categories: red light, yellow light, or green light. Foods that continually fail are considered "red-light" foods. These must always be avoided. Red-light foods should be thought of as energetic allergens.

The foods that constantly ping-pong back and forth from pass to fail are "yellow-light" foods. This category of foods must be rotated. *Rotating* specific yellow-light foods, means they shouldn't be consumed more frequently than once or twice a week. Foods such as olive oil and garlic are typical yellow-light foods, but are almost never rotated because they are thought to be such healthy foods. As such, they tend to be overconsumed. I suggest that you find three oils and rotate them. One week use olive oil, the next week use organic canola, and the next week use flaxseed oil.

The foods that pass every time they are tested are "green-light" foods. After several tests indicate a pattern, I suggest you color-code your food charts accordingly with colored markers. Traffic Light Classification allows you to chart what I like to call the patient's Food Map.

Rotation of foods is a very important aspect of the Whole Health system. We must remember that our bodies have evolved through thousands of years of genetic programming. Our ancestors ate indigenously and seasonally. They ate only what could be grown or found in their local environment. Their dietary rotations were limited by what the seasons and weather patterns dictated. Thus, while our genetic maps are designed for food rotation, our modern ability to transport and preserve food interferes with our natural genetic programming. The Whole Health System has confirmed this to be a key reason for the growing presence of digestive inflammatory conditions such as irritable bowel syndrome, type 2 diabetes, gallbladder disease, and Crohn's disease. Once you have pass/fail tested your subject's food allergies, it's time to pulse test them for their foods.

Pulse Testing Foods—If a food passes for your partner, it is important for them to know just how positive an influence that food has on them. Likewise, if a food fails, it is important for your partner to know just how detrimental that food is for them. Like vital organ pulse testing, food pulse testing is also based on a plus/minus 1–10 score.

Let's say your subject's arm grew weak when you exposed them to a test vial of wheat or simply called out the word *wheat*. They just failed wheat. Keep in mind, this is a straight pass/fail test, but to what degree is wheat potentially compromising their health? Pulse testing allows you to test the specific degree of energetic negativity wheat poses for them.

Inform your partner that you are about to pulse test to learn just how detrimental wheat is for them, from minus 1 to minus 10, with minus 1 being the least detrimental and minus 10 being the most. Call out numbers from minus 1 to minus 10 as you simultaneously pulse-push on their arm after each counted number. If their arm drops at minus 1, it represents the least sensitivity to wheat. If their arm holds strong until the minus 10 is called out, it represents the greatest degree of negative reaction to wheat.

What the pass/fail testing technique initiates is enacted by the EMT pulse testing technique. If you decide not to employ vial testing, "call out" testing will suffice. Your partner's unconscious sixth sense will easily adapt to these changes, provided that you clearly and audibly state the intention of the pulse testing. It takes the unconscious mind only seven-tenths of a second to adapt its neural feedback response.

EMT Food Combination Testing—Over the years, there have been many studies substantiating the validity of proper food combining. Dr. Herbert M. Shelton compiled more than fifty-three years of research data on the topic (between 1928 and 1981). Dr. Shelton's research was first noted by Dr. Philip Norman, in the *Journal of the American Medical Association,* in 1924. Norman also supported the theory of proper food combining, often citing its validity as a science.

The concepts of proper food combining are very simple. The theory is that one should not combine proteins like meat, fish, dairy, eggs, beans, and legumes with starches like potatoes, bread, pasta, and grains. Proteins combine well, however, with low-starch vegetables like broccoli, green beans, spinach, and salads. Fruits should be taken alone, between meals, and if eaten as a fruit salad, combined only within their own groups—acid, subacid, sweet, and melons. So, what's the point of all this?

First, all foods have varying degrees of density. For example, a cut of prime rib is denser than a green bean, and cheese is denser than an apple. Varying degrees of density result in different times necessary for digestion and absorption. Next, when it comes to digestion, proteins, carbohydrates, and fats all perform different tasks. Proteins provide building and repair, while carbohydrates provide fuel and fats as stored energy. Not every human being executes each of these tasks with equal efficiency. For example, those who are diabetic or hypoglycemic tend not to digest and/or assimilate carbohydrates efficiently, while those with gout tend to struggle with protein digestion.

The Whole Health EMT system adds yet another consideration when it comes to proper food combining. Not all food energies combine well with the energies of individual people. The Whole Health system is truly customized to the individual. It offers one the opportunity to utilize the medicinal properties of foods at their maximum potential. I recommend the EMT Food Combining protocol only for those who are extremely sick or terminally ill.

This procedure is easy. Once again, assume the tuning posture. By now your partner has already been fully pass/fail food tested, so simply call out possible food combinations and strength test your partner for each one. For example, call out "Red meat with potatoes" and test their strength. Next call out "Red meat, potatoes, and green beans," and strength test them again. Remember, your unconscious minds are employing the sixth sense, and your electromagnetic fields are relaying the energetic response through your nervous systems and muscles. I always remind my students and patients that I have observed the accuracy and reliability of this sixth-sensory energy system for more than three decades. Your mind/body knows the answer!

Testing for Raw Versus Cooked Food—The question of raw versus cooked food has become a debate of epic proportion. The raw food advocates remind us that enzymes are the vital catalysts of life force and abundant health. The cooked food advocates suggest that the spleen and lymph system function more efficiently with warm, cooked foods. Who is right? Whole Health says they can be both right and wrong, depending on the circumstances and for different people. Whole Health is a system that ascribes to energetic individuality. We are comprised of a myriad of subtle energies and we are all very different, as well as ever changing! Whole Health therefore suggests that the question of raw versus cooked food be individually tested and retested each season. As the seasons change, we change. Simply use the EMT pass/fail (yes/no) testing technique. Hold up your partner's arm and test their strength response when calling out "Cold, raw food" and "Warm, cooked food." You will end the great debate in a swift moment!

EMT Meal Plan Testing—One of the most important EMT protocols is meal plan testing. This is where you can provide your partner with their very own customized diet plan with the optimal recommendations for specific foods and for amounts to be taken at each meal throughout the day. You can even test for how long they are to implement such a diet before it requires updating, as is often necessary, especially during seasonal changes.

Once again, assume the tuning position. Now simply strength test your subject for their daily meals, one meal at a time. Then, muscle test them for each food category at the top of the page. Finally, call out the amounts of each positive food in ounces and muscle test your partner's strength reaction to each amount. For example, call out "Breakfast." Then call out the words *protein, vegetables, fruits,* and *high-starch* carbohydrates. Next call out amounts for whichever foods passed at breakfast. If protein passed, then call out "Three ounces" and strength test them, "Four ounces" and strength test them, and so on. As soon as you find a strong breakfast food and amount, mark it down on your chart. Test for all meals, foods, and amounts until their EMT Meal Plan Map is completed. Last but not least, test them for how long this diet plan is to be adhered to in terms of weeks. Retest their meal plan at that time.

EMT Food Supplement Testing—Nutritional supplements have become an important part of American life. According to the CDC, approximately 50 percent of all Americans take nutritional supplements on a daily basis. That means that millions of Americans are

Prepare a blank meal plan chart that looks something like this:

	PROTEIN	VEGETABLES/FRUITS	HIGH STARCHES
BREAKFAST			
AM SNACK			
LUNCH			
PM SNACK			
DINNER			
EVENING SNACK			

consuming nutritional supplements every day, but few have a solid basis for determining whether what they are choosing to take is in their best interest. Whole Health reminds us that, no different from "potentially" healthy foods, food supplements may actually deplete one's energy. The EMT Food Supplement Testing protocol offers one a customized approach to zeroing in on the safest, most energizing food supplements.

Before you begin this procedure, make a comprehensive list of vitamins, minerals, antioxidants, herbal, and homeopathic supplements they currently take, or may appear to need. (Appendix A presents the entire Whole Health Apothecary of nutritional supplements.) At the top of the page, create four categories: Potency, Dose, Frequency, and Duration. Your list might look something like this:

	POTENCY	DOSE	FREQUENCY	DURATION
VITAMIN A				
VITAMIN C				
CALCIUM				
GINGER				
KALI CARBONICUM				
OTHER				

Now, once again interface with your partner, assuming the proper position. Then muscle test them in a pass/fail manner for each supplement on your list. Following pass/fail testing, you will pulse test your partner for each food supplement. It's only essential to test them for the positive food supplements that they've already passed. As with foods, pulse test them from 1 to 10. Verbally announce your intention to test the positive food supplements in degrees from 1 to 10, and then begin.

The Whole Health protocol recommends that they be instructed to take only those nutritional supplements that pulse higher than five. Anything less than that is simply not worth taking as a supplement. Another note: if you wish to pulse test the negative numbers for those food supplements that failed the pass/fail test, feel free to do so. It can be helpful to demonstrate to your subject that a nutritional supplement they have been taking may actually be depleting their energy. It may make them feel better to stop taking it! Once again, as Whole Health reminds us, one size doesn't fit all! Everyone assumes that all nutritional supplements are good for everybody. When it comes to getting a nutritional supplement plan right for each individual, EMT enables us to thread the needle. That is exactly what you are going to do next.

It's time to begin testing each of your partner's passed nutritional supplements for potency, dose, frequency, and duration. Simply call out the questions and muscle test for each question. Let's take vitamin C, for example. Call out doses beginning with 500 milligrams and test their muscle strength. Call out higher potencies until the arm drops. Find the highest potency that produces a strong muscle response. This represents proper potency for them.

Next, call out doses, or the number of times per day they take their properly dosed vitamin C. Call out "Once a day" and test, then "Twice a day," and test, and so on, until their arm drops. Find the highest number of times that produces a strong muscle response. This represents the proper dose.

Now the number of days per week the vitamin C supplements are to be taken is tested in the same manner. Strength test your partner as you call out, "One day per week," "Two days per week," and so on, testing after each, until you arrive at the most days per week that produces a strong muscle response. This represents the optimal frequency for taking each of their supplements.

Finally, you test your subject for duration: the length of time your partner will remain on this particular nutritional supplement protocol. Simply call out and strength test them for one week, two weeks, three weeks, one month, and so on, until you arrive at the highest number of weeks that produces a strong muscle response. This represents the long-term duration of their nutritional supplement protocol. Duration often manifests in cycles. In other words, sometimes the entire protocol will test positively for a month or so, but the subject may need a week or two off, and then begin a new supplement cycle. An example of a duration cycle may be one that lasts for, say, eight weeks followed by a two-week period of rest from the nutritional supplement. This cycle of eight weeks on and two weeks off may continue repeating ad infinitum, or it may need to be altered at some point. This can all be asked aloud and muscle tested.

Qigong Testing Your Foods and Supplements—By now, you are all tested up and balanced. If you are a bit upset at having to avoid some of your favorite foods because you learned that they either drain or overcharge your energy, fear not. A number of years ago, a friend of mine who is a Chinese master asked me to give a presentation with him at a seminar. He called for several volunteers to come forward. He then asked me to test them for several foods and teas. Next, he asked me to set aside a box of tea that one woman had a very weak reaction to. He then grabbed the box of tea and began moving his hands and his thoughts in a manner intended to infuse the tea with energy. He had an intense, determined look on his face. His mental intention to inject energy into that box of tea was ever clear. His hands kept throwing energy into the box, similar to a chef throwing grains of salt into a skillet. In effect, he was demonstrating how a beverage/food that was devoid of energy for a given person could be infused with energy by performing Qigong (an energy mastery exercise) on that particular food or beverage. Following his energy boost on the box of tea, he asked me to retest her. She passed with flying colors! It was an important lesson about the ways of energy for all in attendance. Energy is everywhere, and it can be dramatically altered with strong mental intention.

The Two Secondary EMT Applications

1. *Testing the Four Energy Quadrants*—There are two additional short-form EMT procedures that support the process of assessment. The first of these is Testing the Four Energy Quadrants (see Figure 4.6). Remember, energy is not only generated and absorbed within the body's internal glands and organs—energy is also collected all around the body's outer field. Outer-field energies are generally derived from all the positive and negative influences around you. By testing the quadrants first, you can establish the energy state of the external body.

   This is a relatively simple test. First assume pass/fail position. Next the practitioner should simply place their free hand in the direction of the subject's upper-right quadrant. The motioning of the practitioner's free hand in this upper-right quadrant is a way of asking the subject's field if there is sufficient energy present in that quadrant. If the subject's arm drops, it means there's a deficiency in that quadrant. Then, repeat this procedure in sequence for the upper-left, lower-left, and lower-right quadrants. If the subject's arm drops while testing any of these quadrants, it indicates a deficiency. This test initiates the Whole Health EMT diagnostic process by determining the energy deficiencies in the outer body field.

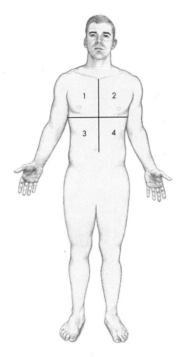

FIGURE 4.6   *The Four Energy Quadrants*

1. The upper-right quadrant reflects the outer-field energy strength of the right lung, liver, and gallbladder.
2. The lower-right quadrant: right kidney and adrenal glands.
3. The upper-left quadrant: left lung and spleen.
4. The lower-left quadrant: left kidney and adrenal glands.

2. *Finger Zone Organ Testing*—The second EMT short-form assessment technique is called finger zone organ testing. Most ancient energy healing systems place great emphasis on the hands and feet, as it is believed that their respective nerve endings correspond with the same nerve networks as all the vital glands and organs. Chinese medicine generally correlates the hands and feet with the meridians of the small intestines, heart, pericardium, large intestine, and lungs. The Korean Koryo Sooji Chim system

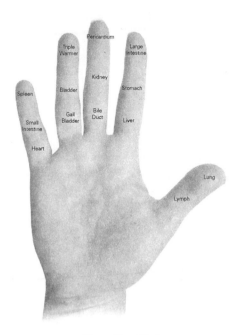

FIGURE 4.7   *Finger Zone Testing*

of hand acupuncture links the hands with virtually every part of the human anatomy. Similarly, the Ayurvedic system of reflexology links the hands and fingers, feet, and toes with all of the vital glands and organs. Whole Health EMT hand zone organ testing is an accurate, simple, short form of diagnostic muscle testing that works very effectively. The Whole Health EMT System of hand/organ mapping between individual finger phalanges and specific organs has been repeatedly tested for pinpoint accuracy.

The human hand has fourteen phalanges—three sections for each finger and two for each thumb. Each section of every finger corresponds energetically with a vital organ (see Figure 4.7). The simple procedure requires the practitioner to muscle test the subject's arm strength while applying light pressure to (pinching) each of the subject's phalanges, one at a time. Anytime the arm drops with sudden loss of energy strength, it signifies deficient energy in the corresponding organ.

The Two EMT Self-Testing Forms

1. *Grasping the Ch'i*—I am often asked if it is possible to pulse test oneself in the absence of a partner. The answer is a resounding "Yes!" I call this technique Grasping the Ch'i. Although not an actual muscle-testing technique, Grasping the Ch'i does require considerable skill and energy sensitivity. The way it works is really quite simple.

Keep in mind that when muscle testing, you are engaging in a biofeedback technique that analyzes the human body's energy field via the neuromuscular system. Anytime we think of anything, either positive or negative, our nervous system is responding at subtle levels that we are not generally tuned in to. These same subtle neurological responses we produce when thinking about good things or bad things may be felt in the palms of our hands. When thinking about something positive or affirmative, there is a light pitter-patter, like light raindrops, in the palm of each hand. When thinking about anything negative, on the other hand, there is no response in the palms at all, just a dead feeling. The Chinese recognized this pitter-patter of neurological excitement in the hand as the movement of ch'i, or life force.

As with all our previous energy protocols, Grasping the Ch'i begins with tuning. Begin by rubbing both palms together vigorously, thirty times. This activates the energy in the palms. Next, close your eyes and think about a positive reference, such as the phrase *I am powerful*. Now draw all your attention to the palms of your hands and try feeling the light pitter-patter of energy. Try several times to Grasp the Ch'i. You may also try focusing on other positive words, phrases, or images. You might try picturing in your mind someone you love very much. Once you have successfully Grasped the Ch'i, you must then experience the difference—the absence of ch'i.

Once again, with eyes closed and palms facing up and open,

think of a negative word, phrase, or image. As you do, feel the clearing out, or absence, of ch'i in your palms. As with the positive exercise, make several attempts. Note the distinct difference between the presence and absence of life force in your palms. Grasping the Ch'i should be considered a pass/fail test. If you become accomplished, you may also master the art of pulse counting while grasping.

2. *Punch-Pushing the Fist*—Grasping the Ch'i demands a great deal of personal ch'i to be effective. A much easier method of EMT self-testing is Punch-Pushing the Fist. I have seen a number of techniques that suggest testing finger strength and leaning forward and backward, but I feel they have very poor reliability. The Punch-Pushing technique is a simple and reliable pass/fail technique that seems to work very well and can be effectively performed while standing or seated.

First, make a taut fist with your nondominant hand. Then, with elbow bent, place your fist directly in front of your heart, approximately two inches away from your chest. Now call out your contrasting positive and negative tuning words or images. Be sure to tune for as long as you need to. It is important to establish a baseline for your testing. Once you are properly tuned, begin calling out the vital organs one at a time and, as you do, try pushing on your fist with your dominant hand. Make sure you push firmly and quickly. Be sure to reset your nondominant hand in place with a taut firmness after each test. A failed response should result in the nondominant fist being easy to push into the chest. Don't make it too difficult for yourself. Simply give in if you sense a natural failed response. This is generally a reliable self-testing technique that you can improve upon easily. You can pass/fail test organs and foods with this technique. As with all these EMT procedures, it is important to practice, practice, practice!

AFTERWARD: EMT ASSESSED AND BALANCED FOR LONGEVITY

Now that you're assessed and balanced, it's time for your ch'i to be preserved. By the preservation of ch'i I'm referring to longevity. Whole Health can put you in a position to cultivate far greater longevity. Let's take a closer look.

The outer membrane of a cell is responsible for transporting oxygen and nutrients to all other parts of that cell. Therefore, nature designed cells to be microscopic is size so as to allow for an efficient delivery of nourishment throughout the cell. The outer cell membrane grows faster than the innermost part of the cell and, as the cells get larger, the outer membrane is then unable to reach all parts of the innermost cell with replenishment. Therefore the cell must go through its natural life cycle until it ultimately divides. Healthy human cells engage in cell division approximately fifty times throughout the span of their duration. Chromosomes are vital to this process, as they contain all the cell information that enables cells to divide. Every time cells divide, their chromosomes get worn down, and aging is the result of this wearing down. But nature offers some protection from the wear and tear of chromosomal aging. The ends of chromosomes are protected by proteins called telomeres. Think of them as protective plastic shoelace caps that keep the chromosomes from fraying every time the cell divides. The shorter our telomeres, the faster we age.

Research has recently discovered a longevity enzyme called telomerase. Telomerase enzymes protect and repair the telomeres, actually extending their length, and thereby reversing the aging process. Longer telomeres are now widely considered to be one of the most reliable anti-aging determinants.

Remember, it's impossible to change your genes more than one-tenth of 1 percent every 250 generations. But you can change the behavior of your genes very easily. Telomerase production is a great example of this, and scientists have discovered a number of behavioral, dietary, and other treatment factors that increase telomerase production.

Donor antioxidants like vitamins A, C, and E have been shown to dramatically increase telomerase by fending off free-radical vampire cells in search of electrons from healthy cells. The vitamins accomplish this by donating their own electrons. Missionary antioxidants like L-glutathione and N-acetyl-cysteine have demonstrated the ability to convert damaging free radical molecules back into antioxidants. The Mediterranean Diet of fish, poultry, vegetables, fruits, and whole grains has been shown to extend telomeres. The story is no different when it comes to natural relaxation response research.

In 2010, a team of German scientists found that fit, active subjects consistently demonstrated 40 percent greater telomere length when compared to their sedentary counterparts. A number of studies have consistently found that dedicated meditators have on average a one-third greater telomere length than nonmeditators.

The ancient Chinese embraced the philosophy of *Mi Bing*, or "Before Disease." Mi Bing reflects their concept of longevity. Keep in mind that they believed that natural human life expectancy was designed to be 120 years. The reason for their focus on self-preservation was to enable the higher self-cultivation of wisdom to better prepare for the next life. This extended cultivation of balance, health, and higher consciousness was tantamount to attaining immortality in their view. Thus, Mi Bing—from the standpoint of disease prevention and longevity—was very important to their concepts of both mortal and immortal life.

The ancients believed that one of the most important ways to engage Mi Bing was to stimulate the Stomach 36 acupuncture point. This point is located one finger width laterally from the anterior border of the tibia (see Figure 4.8). This vital point is said to

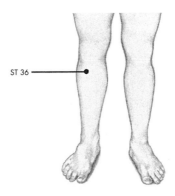

ST 36

FIGURE 4.8   Stomach 36

assist with everything from low immunity and chronic illness to depression and anxiety.

Stomach 36 is considered to be one of the most important of all acupuncture points for the general maintenance and fortification of overall mind/body health. The Chinese name for this point is *Zusanli,* or "Leg Three Miles." During ancient times, people in China traveled mostly on foot, and stimulation of this point was said to relieve fatigue in such a way that, when one hit the point of peak exhaustion, they could then get three more miles out of their tired legs.

The ancients were pretty clear about the life extension properties of Stomach 36, but could this power point actually be a modern-day telomere extender? In his book *The Biophysics for Acupuncture and Health,* Dr. Shui Yin Lo writes of a study that found that acupuncture stimulation of Stomach 36 showed an average increase in telomere length up to two times their length prior to treatment, further citing increases ranging from 60 percent to 100 percent!

Whole Health has adopted a simple plan to diagnose and balance one's longevity energy via Stomach 36.

EMT Longevity Test—Practitioners should begin by once again interfacing with subjects. As with all EMT protocols, first engage in the tuning exercise. Then move onto EMT pass/fail testing while applying light pressure on the subject's Stomach 36 point. For advanced practitioners, touch testing will not be necessary. Simply draw upon strong intention while calling out "Stomach 36." This is all that will be necessary to get effective pass/fail results.

Next, practitioners must initiate the pulse testing procedure. Following the pass/fail test, you'll need to know the degree of strength or weakness of the subject's Stomach 36. As always, pulse testing is a search for a plus/minus factor between 1 and 10. "Minus" represents deficiency and "plus" represents excess or inflammation. If a deficiency is found, then it must be balanced by adding ch'i. This chapter deals exclusively with EMT energy diagnosis. The following chapter on body balancing reveals how to stimulate Stomach 36 to enhance longevity.

Note: It is possible for some subjects to have an excess of energy at Stomach 36. If practitioners discover excess energy at Stomach 36, they should opt instead for Kidney 1, or *Yang Quan,* "Bubbling Spring." This is a very good backup longevity point.

CHAPTER 5

WHOLE HEALTH BODY BALANCING

INFINITE MIND: THE MEDIUM FOR BALANCING THE BODY

As with light, your thought travels through the ether by means of waves that continually extend ever outward. Therefore, your thoughts are "virtual particles," and can, according to the theories of quantum entanglement, simultaneously occupy space in an infinite number of potential locations. This ability of your thoughts to "skip" across domain gaps is referred to as "quantum tunneling."

Thoughts are energy that produces field-generating waves, which travel through space similar to quanta (discrete light packets). Every thought is part of an infinite web of "lightlike" packets that exist everywhere simultaneously. The multiverse is like an information matrix where thought vibrations are transmitted through ether without restriction.

Neurologically, your thoughts travel from your brain to anywhere within your body at the approximate speed of 250 miles per hour. The outer transmission of your thoughts into the ether of space, however, is believed by some experts to travel faster than the speed of light (186,000 miles per second/700 million mph), as they circle the globe more than seven and a half times per second, ad infinitum. Moreover, each of our conscious and unconscious 300 to 3,000 thoughts per minute is enjoined as part of an exponentially expanding collective unconscious and consciousness field. We're all being affected concurrently by the resonance of each other's thoughts.

Imagine someone thousands of miles away transmitting thought patterns that you're unconsciously receiving. What influence might those thoughts have on your mood, your behaviors, and the outcome of your day? What about your wishes, hopes, and dreams? They are also thoughts that are influencing other thinkers, even as you read this. How much of what is currently in your life was magnetically brought in by your past thoughts? Can you bring new, more advantageous people and circumstances into your life by thinking more aligned thoughts? Most of us believe that we are affected only by those thoughts within and immediately around us, but we're all continually being affected by the thoughts of many distant thinkers, perhaps even from universes and worlds beyond. What's more, this process of thought field transmission is far from random.

Vibrations are oscillations of energy waves that are both transmitted and received. Vibratory wave patterns find their way to compatible or energetically matched vibratory receptors. Most believe that their thoughts travel but a very short distance, only to swiftly dissipate into the ether. But this is simply not so. Every single thought emitted finds its way to sympathetic vibratory receptors here, there, and everywhere. The truth is, thought travel is not finite nor is its transit random. Every thought vibration transmitted is received by like vibrations. Thought travel is governed by the law of attraction. Energies that vibrate at the same frequency are magnetically drawn to each other. The feelings that inspire our thoughts influence their vibratory nature. For example, inspired thoughts of spiritual love are defined and empowered by their spiritual and emotional intentions. They are driven by powerful energies that magnetically shuttle them to their similar destinations. Thoughts are things—powerful things—and they travel infinite distances, ultimately arriving in an instant exactly where they were intended to go. Thoughts have great power.

DISTANT HEALING THOUGHTS

Local medicine is constructed on an antiquated foundation. The inescapable physics by which nonlocal or distance healing derives self-evidence has at last begun to surface. Over the past thirty years, there have been hundreds of distance prayer and healing studies, including some performed at respected institutions of higher learning such as Dartmouth College, Duke University Medical Center, and the University of California School of Medicine in San Francisco. Most of this research has produced evidence supporting the argument for nonlocal healing efficacy, supporting the argument that thought indeed travels through space in an ordered fashion.

There are theorists who've attempted to explain distance telepathy and healing prayer from the perspective of quantum mechanics. "Zero-point field" is a term for a quantum vacuum state containing no physical particles. It is believed to contain virtually no energy. It would be a mistake, however, to think of this field as an empty state, as it contains an infinite amount of fleeting electromagnetic waves and particles that continuously "pop" in and out of existence and can be influenced by the mere act of observation. Many argue that zero-point field allows for manipulation in the space-time continuum via scalar waves. The scalar waves that zero-point field generates represent a quantum theory that opens doors to an array of infinite possibilities, including an explanation for the nonrandom nature of distance communication.

While all this conjecture attempted to logically and scientifically explain the mechanics of distance communication and healing over the past several decades (and took its time in doing so), I've managed to help thousands of people around the country and world with the power of distance healing thoughts. I decided long ago to leave the debating to others. I simply wanted to explore the possibility of healing anyone I could, regardless of how far away they were.

Initially, I just wanted to take some time to get comfortable with the process, and to establish whether I could indeed have a healing effect nonlocally. Straightaway, the feedback I received made it clear that there was something very real and very special taking place. Almost immediately, most of those who I worked with at distances informed me of swift and dramatic improvements. As I mentioned earlier, headaches were frequently relieved during the course of a phone call. Many of the acute pain and inflammation cases I worked with were aided within a week's time. I must admit, I was stunned. I hadn't expected to see such swift, remarkable results. My nonlocal healing work took off overnight as I suddenly found myself fielding numerous national and global referrals from the people I was able to assist.

Based on my own empirical evidence I can now say, without hesitation, that I believe distant thoughts can effectively be transmitted to any distant domain by the power of healing intention.

One of my earliest experiences with distance Wenchiech'u healing (a concept that will be fully explored later in this chapter) was with a young man from California who was injured in a surfing accident some years earlier. He had been violently knocked off of his board by the wild Pacific surf and managed to come away with only minor injuries, but still suffered chronic dull pain in his lower back that no one was able to help him with. He tried a number of prescriptive and over-the-counter medications, as well as nutritional supplements, to no avail. He'd also undergone extensive physical therapy, but saw no improvement.

We had a brief telephone consult and I asked him about the status of his general health prior to the accident. He conveyed that he was in good health except for a recurrent problem with urinary tract infections. He told me he had averaged at least three or four per year. My study of Chinese medicine alerted me to the fact that the psoas muscle (which was the source of his pain) is energetically connected to the kidneys. I immediately suspected that a chronic kidney deficiency was at the root of both his urinary tract infections as well as his current lower-back pain.

We scheduled a follow-up telephone appointment in one week, and immediately after hanging up the phone I began directing healing counterclockwise spirals to his deficient kidneys. I transmitted a series of these Wenchiech'u exercises at two-minute intervals. I performed two-minute boosters once daily for three days. On the fourth day I was surprised and pleased to hear that for the first time in five years, his lower-back pain had at last subsided. Nearly a year later he called to inform me that he'd had one full year without any urinary tract infections.

I continue to effectively perform many nonlocal healing sessions for patients from all around the world. I can now personally testify to the fact that the quantum power of the mind has remarkable healing powers, and that conscious positive intentions do indeed find their way to exactly where they belong. I also believe that whatever positive conscious intentions I transmit in the form of thought are received not just by the person I am working with, but by whomever else they might resonate with, anywhere in the multiverse, at any time.

THOUGHT BEYOND SPACE AND TIME

Recently, I delivered four seminars within ten days of each other, the last of which marked my five hundredth public speaking event. For more than half of those seminars and lectures, I've demonstrated one particular group-distance healing experiment that has never failed to deliver. I begin by calling up a volunteer. After a few brief formalities, I immediately begin muscle testing the subject's organ strengths and weaknesses. I test their arm strength resistance with one hand, while placing mild pressure on the various organ pressure points of their body with the other hand. As soon as the volunteer's arm drops upon discovery of an organ deficiency, we stop. I then ask for the audience to help us. I instruct them to focus their healing intention on the subject's area of weakness.

In this case, my subject displayed a very weak muscle response when I applied light pressure to her Lung 1 acupuncture point, just below the clavicle. So the audience was asked to focus the power of their healing attention on the subject's clavicle. They were then asked to envision themselves as transmitting a laser-like light of healing energy from their minds directly to her deficient clavicle,

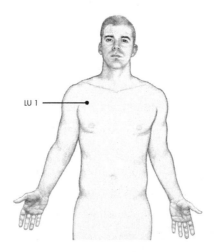

LU 1

FIGURE 5.1 *Lung 1*

with the express intention of strengthening her deficient lung energy. After ninety seconds of audience distance healing, I retested the subject's Lung 1 strength. And, just as it has happened hundreds of times before, the subject's arm suddenly showed no weakness. I always tell them that we just took a walk on the edge of physics, where together we suspended the notion of time and space. Sound a bit like theater?

All meaning previously assigned to the concepts of time and space is becoming problematic. Ever since Einstein's general and special theories of relativity were first postulated more than a century ago, the concept of time and space as constants has, in essence, been greatly diminished. Time and space have assigned relative value only in our material world. As Einstein reminds us, "Time and space are modes by which we think, and not conditions in which we live."

The phenomenon of "retrocausation" obliterates all boundaries associated with the concept of time. This concept suggests that the future can affect the present, and the present can affect the past. Retrocausation serves as a reminder that there are no laws governing the direction of what we perceive as time flow. What we perceive as time doesn't just move forward, but in all directions simultaneously.

Garret Moddel, a professor of electrical engineering at the University of Colorado (Boulder), has spoken extensively on the connection between retrocausation and the laws of entropy. Like much of the existing psychokinetic research, Moddel posits that, based on the second law of thermodynamics (i.e., the disorder in a system always increases and never decreases), the degree of a subject's energy is consistent with the likelihood of such an event occurring. In other words, the greater the subject's emotion, the greater the likelihood of recognizing a retrocausation response. Moddel also points to what's called the bilking paradox, an assertion that shatters causality by substituting free will in place of the functionality of time and space. It firmly centers its relative basis for reality within the observer's perception. Moddel asserts that there has been more than enough sufficient experimental evidence that has evolved from logic to modeling to support retrocausality.

Princeton University physicist and researcher York Dobyns has performed a number of published experiments on humans with devices that have tested the paranormal realm of possibility far beyond the human senses. More recently, Dobyns completed experiments where human operators were able to consistently analyze and alter events retroactively through intention at distances. Dobyns's most recent retrocausation study was published in the *Journal of Scientific Exploration* in 2011. To date there are twenty-six meta-analysis reviews showing statistical significance regarding retrocausation.

Yet, while we know retrocausation exists, no one really knows the mechanics behind it. Some suggest that quantum mechanics might best explain the phenomenon. The laws of quantum mechanics suggest that there need not be a prior rationale for any event—rather, events can, and do, often exhibit a random nature. In this sense, retrocausation may be thought of as a sort of Lorentz transformation variant—that is, a special relativity whereby events of space and time are measured and based not on absolutes, but rather, on the relative perceptions of observers. The quantum perspective on retrocausation may reveal reflections of what Einstein called "spooky action at a distance" (where there is nonlocal interaction between objects beyond the limitations of time and space) or "superposition" (objects are in all states simultaneously, as long as they're not limited by observation) or "quantum entanglement" (where the states of two or more objects, while individual and spatially separated, remain interactive).

As it is perceived in our world, time only seems to move forward. But the truth of the matter is that time isn't governed by laws that restrict it from moving backward. Researcher Ferenc Krausz of the Max Planck Institute for Quantum Optics in Germany has clocked the shortest time intervals ever recorded. The events he observes are a reflection of the temporal-time world known as the Planck scale, which deals in the smallest units of time. The fastest motions in the microscopic world produce near-infinitesimal times. Krausz has recorded times in the "attoseconds." A nanosecond is a billion times faster than a second, and an attosecond is another billion faster than a nanosecond. Krausz's work is on the brink of breaking the barrier of time as we know it. The barrier of space is about to be breached as well.

John Cramer, a well-known and respected physicist at the University of Washington, believes that light particles can work in reverse. He refers to his theory as the "transactional interpretation of quantum mechanics." Cramer emphasizes that there is no proof that time can move only one way, and no logical explanation why it can't work backward. He is in the process of proving his theory with the aid of lasers, prisms, splitters, and fiber optics. His experiment intends to demonstrate signaling between entangled light particles in reverse time.

TRANSMITTING THOUGHT CH'I

The quantum physics of the modern West and the alchemy of the ancient East share one very important commonality—an understanding of energy. While quantum physics has come to better understand energy through analytical and theoretical analysis, ancient Eastern alchemy demands a purely innate understanding of energy. Nonetheless, each of these divergent perspectives opens us up to the limitless potentials of energy.

Like atoms, there will never be a shortage of ch'i. Remember that ch'i manifests in an endless myriad of forms, including thought. Therefore, energy healing is a matter of effectively directing thought ch'i to wherever there is a perceived deficiency. This is called *Qigong*, or "energy mastery." With Qigong, the life force energy of ch'i can be transmitted from one mind to another regardless of apparent time and space limitations. That is where the practitioner and their intent comes into play. A capable practitioner can artfully channel ch'i from one place to another. They might direct their own ch'i to a patient in need, or they might direct ch'i from out of the air, sun, stars, skies, or rain. A good practitioner might visualize a waterfall or a rainbow in their mind as a source of ch'i to be directed to a subject. They might also recall a wonderful energizing event from their past from which to draw energy for channeling.

I often remind my patients that ch'i is the energetic currency of change. Everything is ch'i, and everything can therefore be altered through the intentional rearrangement of its ch'i. A powerful intention can weaken a virus or strengthen a kidney. Foods and medicines can be energetically altered as well. If a patient has a sinus problem and happens to have a homeopathic for stomachache, I will intentionally alter the energetic properties of their homeopathic medicine to be able to assist with their sinus problem. Homeopathy has very active ch'i, powerful receptor energy, and memory that can be intentionally reprogrammed with the power of positive-thought ch'i.

Body balancing between a practitioner and subject begins with two very important prerequisites: 1) the practitioner must have powerful intention to heal the subject, and 2) the subject must be open to receiving the healing ch'i. If either of these elements is absent, the healing will likely not be successful. Energy healing with ch'i is a form of thought communication. There must be a transmitter and a receiver, or there can be no effective two-way connection. When it comes to transmitting healing-thought ch'i, there are two prerequisite healing-thought intentions.

The Two Prerequisites for Transmitting Thought Ch'i

1. Loving Compassion (yin)
2. Healing Determination (yang)

While either one alone will be sufficient, the ideal situation is for the practitioner to have both intentions within command. Healing compassion is not an easy thing for most people to cultivate in today's competitive world. I always believed that it was a good exercise for any healing practitioner to connect with the face of innocence and deservedness. By observing children at play, or the elderly with their limitations, or the handicapped with their challenges, it becomes easier to connect with innocence and deservedness. The next step of course is to transmit the ch'i generated by these visions to the subject you wish to heal. Regardless of what we appear to be, our core forever remains the same. Life is hard. Pain and suffering are strangers to no one. It's important for all practitioners to tap into their wellspring of compassion and learn to transmit the ch'i it generates.

The power of our compassion may be best exemplified by the Buddhist practice of compassion meditation. University of Wisconsin neuroplasticity researchers recently studied the brain waves of the Dalai Lama's monks after one of their compassion meditations. Each of the monks was hooked up to 256 electrodes for brain scanning. The researchers were stunned to record gamma brain wave bursts never before recorded by science and not believed capable of being captured. The researchers had expected relaxation, in the form of alpha brain waves. The key thing to take away from this is that their compassion meditation was anything but passive. The power of their intention was more like a World Series pitcher on the mound, focusing only on the catcher's mitt. In a zone so intense, they don't even hear the roar of the 50,000 spectators cheering them on. The monks were in a zone of their own, and just as soon as their eyes closed, they were determined to have a very real, tangible healing effect somewhere in this world. Imagine closing your eyes and having the world in your arms as if it were a wounded child. Think of yourself as creating an intentional and powerful healing energy that was absolutely going to have an effect. Like a practitioner with powerful healing determination, these monks simply won't take no for an answer. There is great healing power in our most compassionate thoughts and intentions.

THE HEART'S HAND

The Heart's Hand is a distance energy healing technique that I discovered while in stream of consciousness during a seminar many years ago. It is the simplest of all body balancing techniques. In the middle of this particular seminar, I requested a volunteer. A gentleman raised his hand and came up to the front of the group. I was demonstrating the pass/fail organ test and found that he had a deficient gallbladder that pulse tested at −6. Prior to the class, I'd spoken with him for a while and our conversation had revealed that he was taking the course to learn to better care for his grandsons, who'd lost their parents. He was the designated caregiver and wanted to learn all he could to better serve the well-being of his grandsons. It was plain to see that he loved those little boys more than life itself. The mere mention of their names evoked great emotion in him. So when it came time to balance his deficient gallbladder, an instinct came over me to ask him to close his eyes, place his hands over his gallbladder, and instead of spiraling, or weaving ch'i, I simply asked the man to envision his grandsons. I asked him to collect the energy of that image and then to direct the love it generated directly to his gallbladder. I asked him to remain concentrated on that vision for a full minute or so. I then retested his gallbladder energy, and of course it was extremely strong. I then tested it again with the pulse test technique to see just how strong it was. After a mere moment or two of ch'i collecting, his gallbladder pulse tested to +10. It was truly remarkable!

This technique greatly inspired everyone in the class. We then attempted a variation on the theme. I asked another volunteer to come forth. Performing the same technique, I discovered that the woman had deficient kidneys that pulsed to −8. This time I asked the class to help out. I instructed the volunteer to place both hands over her primary kidney points, one inch to the right and left of her navel. I then asked each member of the class to think of something or someone they loved very much. I gave them a few moments to collect the ch'i from their visualization. I then asked the woman to close her eyes as the class sent nonlocal, distance love-energy to her kidney area. After a moment or two I retested the volunteer's kidneys and discovered a very strong muscle response. Next, I pulse tested and found that her kidneys had strengthened from −8 to +10. I reminded the class that they had just transmitted collected energy nonlocally, at a distance of some twenty to thirty feet. I asked the class if they believed it was possible for them to produce similar results for subjects at a far greater distance. They all said yes, and their instincts were exactly correct. Such transmission of energy is not restricted by the limitations of time and space. The Heart's Hand exercise is one of the most powerful techniques I have ever worked with. The heart's field of consciousness focuses its attention on a powerful image of love, collects it, and then transmits its great force through the hand of a subject and on to wherever the healing is directed.

WEAVING THE CH'I

The first Whole Health body balancing technique is actually one that has been commonly practiced in China for centuries. It is a Qigong protocol that weaves ch'i into the energy-deficient subject or out of the subject with excess energy. The practitioner will mentally focus on weaving balanced ch'i into any corresponding excess or deficient organs of their subjects with their mind's intention and the movement of their dominant hand. When we speak of the power of the mind's intention, we are really talking about compassion. The practitioner's compassion must be understood as the most

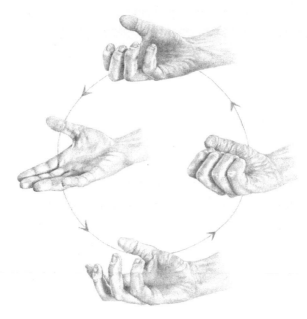

FIGURE 5.2   *Weaving the Ch'i*

important aspect of all Qigong healing. It is compassion that en-gages the "heart-mind." The heart-mind is the ruler of all human life energy.

The technique is quite easy to understand and perform, but it is very powerful. Any subject's organ areas that are deficient will need to have ch'i added, or "weaved in." The practitioner will use their dominant hand to throw ch'i into that weak organ area. This mo-tion is, again, a bit like throwing spice into a cooking pot, but it must be a repeated motion (see Figure 5.2). As with all Qigong healing, the practitioner must focus their mind and envision that they are actually throwing energy into their subject, with the ex-press intention of giving them an energy boost. The practitioner's mental intention means everything. With Qigong, mental intention is what moves the energy. Regardless of the fact that they are inten-sifying their intention, the practitioner isn't giving up their own ch'i, but rather, acting as a medium who is directing the abundant universal ch'i into the subject. This Weaving the Ch'i exercise should take only one to three minutes per organ. Continue to diagnostically pulse test the organ you are working on to see if the organ is balancing. Don't stop treatment until it's balanced.

If your subject has an excess of ch'i, the practitioner must weave the excess energy out of them. When weaving excess ch'i out of a subject, remember to throw it back out into the universe, where it can be cleansed and recycled. Excess ch'i can be energetically toxic. It may represent an accumulated buildup of stress, negative thought emotions, foods, and/or drugs. It may also be the result of bacterial, viral, or fungal infections, electromagnetic pollution, or a number of other causes. Therefore, when performing the Weaving the Ch'i protocol in order to remove excess ch'i, practitioners must occasionally take a moment to shake out any toxic ch'i they might have absorbed.

Practitioners should focus their attention on the subject's area of excess and use their action hand to weave it out and throw it away. Recheck the subject with pulse test diagnostics to see if the organ energy is balancing and, as always, don't stop treatment until you help them to attain balance. As with weaving in, this exercise should take only one to three minutes per organ.

FLUTTERING THE CH'I

This healing Qigong protocol is designed to produce the same results as Weaving the Ch'i *in* and *out*. It employs the same intention but requires a different hand technique. Instead of a weaving motion, the practitioner raises and lowers the hand in a fluttering manner (see Figure 5.3). When married with the mind's intention, the hand becomes a transmitter of energy. That's how energy works. All healing Qigong exercises are most empowered by linking the mind's intention with demonstrative emphasis.

The practitioner must once again focus on the subject's specific

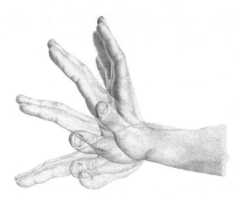

FIGURE 5.3   *Fluttering the Ch'i*

area of organ imbalance. If there is organ deficiency, it calls for fluttering the ch'i upward. For this exercise, I prefer to place my non-dominant hand directly on the deficient organ of focus so as to make a kinetic connection with it. This helps to awaken the energy of the organ. Next, the practitioner must begin engaging their action hand in a fluttering motion as they raise and lower their dominant arm. The emphasis with this motion is both the hand fluttering and the upward raising of the arm.

As always, intention is paramount. The practitioner's mind must focus on the intention to increase the subject's ch'i. They must attempt to synchronize this strong intention with the upward dominant hand fluttering and the dominant arm raising. Weaving and fluttering will never fail to direct the healing ch'i as intended.

WEAVING AND FLUTTERING
THE CH'I NONLOCALLY

In the event that you are trying to balance a subject with the weaving or fluttering techniques at a distance, practitioners will need to use both hands to perform the two balancing exercises described above. The right hand remains the "action" hand. The left hand is what I call the "movie" or "visualization" hand. The key is to visualize the distant subject in the left hand and to generate the ch'i balancing action from the action hand. Make sure to engage an energetic interaction between your two hands. Both weaving and/or fluttering motions must be directed from the right to the left hand. The left hand is representative of the recipient (subject) of the transmitted healing.

When performing these protocols at a distance, one of the most important aspects is the visualization. We are materially programmed to such an extent that many of us have a difficult time with visualizing something that isn't present before us. I am often asked by students what they should be visualizing at a distance during nonlocal healing. Here is a sample of some of the most common questions I have been asked over the years:

- Should we try to visualize the person?
- What if we've never met them?
- Should we try to visualize the organ that we're working in?
- What does a liver look like?
- What if I lose my visual concentration in the middle of the exercise?

My answer is: "Do not worry about your material weaknesses. Instead practice developing your energetic strengths!" It is all about the energy of your intention and the empowerment of your compassion. Fill your movie hand with a generalized picture from your mind's eye of a human being who has experienced great pain, suffering, and confusion. Feel their innocence and their deservedness. Open your heart and let it be drawn to the transcendent power within you that heals. Here there is no need for pictures of people's faces or organs. Here there is only energy that transcends all limitations of time and space. This is not a place of pictures. This is a place of miracles.

SPIRAL POWER

The spiral is a sacred shape that is ever present throughout the natural universe. To the ancients, the spiral symbolized the sacred dance of evolution, the ever-unraveling, infinite birth-to-death continuum. Where the circle represents a continuum that keeps on going around and around, the spiral represents change and new beginnings. According to ancient Ayurvedic and Buddhist traditions, the spiral represents the shape of the chakras, or body centers, where life force is collected. The word *chakra* means "spinning spiral-shaped wheel."

The Ayurvedic culture from India paralleled that of the ancient Chinese when it came to energy mastery. One of the central themes of their energy healing wisdom was that of *Kundalini*, which means "coiled" or "spiral energy." It espouses greater self-realization through yoga, diet, and spiritual discipline, which are believed to result in the ascension of spiraling life-force energy that infuses the body's life-force energy centers (chakras). The higher the spiraling energy rises, the more evolved the individual's consciousness, the more balanced their energy systems, and the greater their overall well-being.

In accordance with the beliefs of Hinduism, Buddhism, Jainism, and Sufism, there are numbers that are sacred. These sacred numbers ultimately arrive at sacred shapes. Spirals—unlike squares, rectangles, and triangles—are open-ended, infinitely extending the potential expression of their shape. All sacred shapes have great power, but none more than the spiral.

The spiral was represented at the birthing of the universe. When proton formations first gathered, following the Big Bang, spiraling particles began swirling and forming energy fields. The positively charged protons moved in a counterclockwise direction and the negatively charged electrons circled in a clockwise direction. The movement of these fundamental particles represents the power and force of spiral motion.

Throughout nature, the spiral is a recurring theme. Examples of the spirals of life can be found everywhere—in the formations of galaxies, the orbiting of planets, hurricanes, tornadoes, the DNA double helix, the umbilical cord, seed patterns (think of the sunflower) and vines, ammonites, and the nautilus and many other shells. Carl Jung referred to the spiral as a symbol of cosmic force.

A MIDSUMMER NIGHT'S DREAM

Many years ago, on a warm summer's eve, I decided to relieve all my workday stresses in the cozy comforts of a lawn chair in my backyard paradise. I distinctly remember putting my head back and gazing up at the radiant glow of luminous starlight, flickering in infinite space. The majesty of it all was awe-inspiring, so much so that I fell asleep in a mere matter of minutes. But it really wasn't just sleep that I fell into. It seemed I had slipped into a trance. My eyes were closed, and I was in a deeply relaxed state, but I almost immediately started having very detailed visions. One vision was of an ancient Chinese man who kept making spiraling motions before me. Over and over, his arms swirled in circular, spiral-like motions. First he swirled his arms and hands clockwise, then counterclockwise. He repeated this over and over. I merely observed confusedly. He had a disturbed look on his face, as if he was growing intemperate with my ignorance. He then began repeatedly showing me images of the T'ai Chi Circle (akin to the yin/yang symbol). As he did, he once again began circling his arms in spiral motions, but this time he did so around the symbol, first in a counterclockwise direction, then in a clockwise direction. He did this for what seemed like an eternity. I pulled myself out of the trance, suddenly came to my senses, and just laughed and shrugged it off.

The next day someone accidentally left in my offices a book entitled *The Chinese Art of T'ai Chi Ch'uan* by Master Chee Soo. I picked it up to have a look. I turned immediately to a page that described an ancient healing art called Wenchiech'u ("thermogenesis"), an ancient healing discipline that balances life-force energy through the artful implementation of spiral energy. Literally translated, *thermogenesis* means "creation of heat."

Traditionally, the practitioner would make spiral motions with their hands ever so lightly on the surface of the subject's skin. This stimulating healing touch was referred to as "contact thermogenesis." The heat generated by contact thermogenesis was believed to circulate the movement of blocked ch'i. Not unlike the other eight healing brocades—acupuncture, acupressure, massage, nutrition, herbal medicine, physical exercise, and meditation—with Wenchiech'u, the goal is to balance the body by unblocking the ch'i.

Following my backyard trance and kismet book discovery, I immediately engaged in further research and study of Wenchiech'u. I also received a great deal more channeled information on the topic, which I adapted through the endless muscle testing Q&A trials. I eventually began developing styles of noncontact Wenchiech'u into my daily work, which enabled me to advance the healing art form nonlocally.

Around that same time, I came to realize that my vision of the T'ai Chi Circle was intended to awaken me to the realization that the Great Circle, while visually static, represents the fluid movement of clockwise and counterclockwise spirals. These motions in turn represent the spiral patterns and movements that balance all universal energies (yin and yang).

As we've discussed, with energy there are only three possible outcomes—excess, deficiency, or balance. If you wanted to stimulate a subject's deficient metabolism, you might assume that they had an energy blockage in their thyroid. Blockages such as this represent an energy deficiency. Blockages and the energy deficiencies they create are classified as "cool or cold." Your intention then would be to stimulate, or strengthen, the thyroid energy by generating "heat." It is important to point out that in classical Chinese medicine, heat is not only a physical, material manifestion; it is also considered a phenomenon of sorts. The kind of heat that they refer to can't always be physically measured. This heat is representative of what they call *Yang Ch'i* or "activating life force energy." The practitioner of Wenchiech'u gains access to the power to either increase or decrease the amount of this heat or life energy in themselves, other people, foods, and environments.

Let's say the food you are about to eat is highly processed and lacking nutrients. It would be considered deficient, and therefore "cooling." If you were adept at Wenchiech'u, you could, in effect, add life force energy to your deficient food, making it healthier for you to consume. Or, if the room you had just entered was hot and stuffy with a crowd of nervous people, you might consider releasing some of the excess energy in the room in order to produce a more comfortable experience. Perhaps you are with a friend who is fighting the flu and is weak, chilled, and fatigued. Your friend is deficient, cool, and in need of warming immune stimulation. To look at your friend in another way, instead of charging up their immune system, you might consider draining the energy out of their virus. My suggestion would be to do both. Charge up their immunity *and* drain the virus. Regardless of whether the practitioner wishes to increase or decrease the ch'i of anyone or anything, Wenchiech'u spirals provide an extremely powerful solution.

WENCHIECH'U PREPARATION EXERCISE

Before beginning body balancing, one should first perform some preparation exercises. In order to effectively transmit healing ch'i with Wenchiech'u, you must energize your vital organ systems by linking them together with light. Our organs perform miracles every day of our life without ever being the focus of our attention. The only time we tend to focus on our organs is when they speak to us in their language of pain. If we are going to ask them to help us generate and transmit healing power, we must first energize them for the task at hand.

This is a simple procedure that one can easily do with or without a partner. Just as it suggests, the intention is to link up the organs with a laser-like beam of white light. You can begin in a seated or standing position.

Linking the Organs with Light:
The Five Elements Vital Organ Cycle

1. *Liver to Heart:* Close your eyes, take three clearing breaths, and relax. Place your right hand over your liver and your left hand over your heart (see Figure 5.4). This initiates the linking of your liver energy with your heart energy. Now envision a laser-like beam of healing *red light* being directed from your right hand (liver) to your left hand (heart). Maintain that intention and vision for approximately two minutes (again, do not worry about timing yourself exactly—concentrate more on the exercise). Now you have light-linked the energy between your liver and heart.

2. *Heart to Spleen:* Next, place your right hand over your heart and your left hand over your spleen. In your mind's eye, visualize a laser-like ray of healing *yellow light* being transmitted from your right hand (heart) to your left hand (spleen). Once again hold the intention and vision for approximately two minutes. Your heart and spleen are now light-linked.

3. *Spleen to Lungs:* Place the right hand over your spleen and your left hand over your lungs. Visualize a *white light* flowing from the right hand (spleen) to your left hand (lungs). Hold the intention and vision for two minutes. Your spleen and lungs are now light-linked.

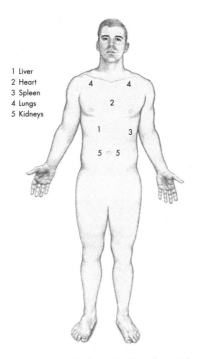

1 Liver
2 Heart
3 Spleen
4 Lungs
5 Kidneys

FIGURE 5.4   Linking the Organs with Light

4. *Lungs to Kidneys:* Place your right hand over your lung and your left hand over your kidney. Picture a *blue light* being sent from your right hand (lungs) to your left hand (kidney). Hold the intention and vision in your mind for two minutes. Your lungs and kidneys are now light-linked.

5. *Kidneys to Liver:* Place your right hand over your kidney and your left hand over your liver. Visualize a beam of healing *green light* passing from your right hand (kidney) to your left hand (liver). Hold the intention and vision for two minutes. Your kidneys and liver are now light-linked.

This completes the Five Elements Vital Organ Cycle. You have now light-linked your vital organs in natural sequence from liver to heart, spleen to lungs, and kidneys to liver.

WENCHIECH'U

Wenchiech'u is the most powerful vehicle for energy balancing that I know of. It has virtually no limitations, and its effectiveness is faultless and time-tested. Powerful healing ch'i produces an energetic type of heat that is very different from the material heat that can be measured. There have been studies where scientists have noted a distinct warming effect produced by ch'i that can actually generate steam.

There are two forms of Wenchiech'u—contact thermogenesis and noncontact thermogenesis. The contact form may only be performed "hands-on," face-to-face. Noncontact Wenchiech'u, on the other hand, may be conducted nonlocally, over any distance. Even though it might seem like a paradox to our Western minds, noncontact or distance Wenchiech'u is much more powerful than the contact form, because energy that is transmitted at a distance masses, or collects energy, as it transits through space.

Wenchiech'u is a form of mental Qigong, which can be translated as "mind energy mastery." Qigong is a 5,000-year-old energy healing discipline, represented by many distinct and varying forms. Generally, Qigong is the alignment of breath, movement, and awareness. However, the two most important elements in effective Qigong practice are willpower and concentration.

Ancient Chinese energy healers clearly understood that everything is energy, even thoughts. Thoughts that carry a powerful intention with intense concentration are among the most powerful manifestations of ch'i, and are most important for generating Qigong power. Similarly, Wenchiech'u demands the willpower of compassion, as well as great mental concentration, in order to be truly effective. So it all begins and ends with the practitioner's mind. Once the waves of concentration and healing intention are deeply set within the mind of the practitioner, Wenchiech'u healing may commence.

Concentration must be fixed on two intentions—to stimulate deficient ch'i and to drain excessive ch'i. Remember, when evaluating energy, there are but three possibilities—excess, deficiency, or balance. The goal of Wenchiech'u is to restore energy balance by adding to the deficiency and subtracting from the excess. There is always a drawstring effect with all ch'i imbalances. That is to say, when one area shifts out of balance due to excess, another corresponding area will become severely deficient.

The goal of the Wenchiech'u treatment will generally depend on the diagnostic energy assessment that preceded it. All the yin and yang organ systems that are deficient should be treated with warming, stimulating, counterclockwise spirals. All the organ systems with excess energy are to be balanced by energy-releasing clockwise spirals. As far as targeting exactly where practitioners are to direct their Wenchiech'u healing spirals, one may simply refer to the Wenchiech'u Treatment Zones charts (see Figure 5.5). These charts map all the major organ reference points. Once the subject's imbalances have been determined, the practitioner may direct Wenchiech'u spirals to the corresponding vital organ areas.

The best way to detect if a treatment is working is to diagnostically pulse test and retest the organ systems that have been treated. If the subject's arm drops, the organ is still deficient and requires more stimulation. If it pulses to a count between eight and ten, it should be considered balanced. If it pulses higher than ten, it is overstimulated and the excess energy should be released.

If the practitioner is in the physical presence of the subject, they can perform contact thermogenesis, which is a "hands-on" practice, either lightly touching the subject or positioning their action hand close to the subject while performing Wenchiech'u. If the subject is at a distance, however, practitioners must direct their noncontact Wenchiech'u intentions and actions nonlocally. Nonlocal Wenchiech'u is transmitted through mental intention from the practitioner's mind to the subject.

Nonlocal Wenchiech'u doesn't always have the benefit of a diagnosis. Therefore, practitioners should at least have a brief discussion with subjects to determine their patterns of imbalance (excess and deficiency). It should be noted here that a practitioner is not essential. One may practice Wenchiech'u on themselves by simply visualizing and directing clockwise and counterclockwise spirals to whatever areas of the body demand it. Here are a few pairs of common excess and deficiency patterns that occur together (see Figure 5.5A):

Excess Energy—Deficient Energy

Virus (CV 7)—Immune system (Thymus Zone)
Allergies (ST 1)—Lymph (Lung Zone)
Anxiety (stress) (PC 8)—Adrenals (Adrenal Medulla Zone)
Acid Reflux (CV 17)—Stomach (Stomach Zone)

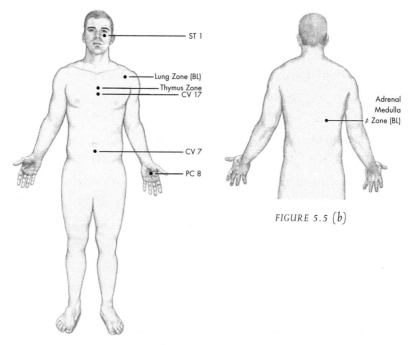

ST 1

Lung Zone (BL)
Thymus Zone
CV 17

Adrenal
Medulla
Zone (BL)

CV 7

PC 8

FIGURE 5.5 (b)

FIGURE 5.5 (a)   Excess/Deficiency Patterns

As one becomes more comfortable thinking about and working with energy, the complexities of excess and deficiency become a matter of common sense. The excess/deficiency chart above points this out. For example, let's look at the first figure—viral excess. Viruses are inflammatory events that generate fevers and heat. Therefore, like all forms of inflammation, viruses are a reflection of excess energy. But viral excess never initiates the imbalance— instead, immune system deficiency does that. Only when the protective immune system is deficient is a virus free to generate its debilitating excess energy. When it comes to viruses, practitioners would do well to spin clockwise spirals at CV 7 to release the excess viral energy and counterclockwise at the Thymus Zone to increase immune energy.

The same holds true for allergies, anxiety, and acid reflux, among other ailments. These conditions reflect inflammation, burning, heat, acidity, and obsessive worry. Clearly they are all representative of excess energy. As with viruses, however, we see a pattern where deficiencies open the door for excesses. For example, allergic inflammation (ST 1) begins with a blocked, deficient lymph system (Lung Zone) that can no longer filter toxins and allergens out of the blood. Similarly, the emotional and mental excesses of anxiety (PC 8) are initiated by acute stresses that exhaust the adrenal glands (Kidney Zone). And the pain and excess inflammation of acid reflux (CV 17) often begin with a severe digestive deficiency (Stomach Zone).

Another diagnostic option is to surrogate test for the subject following a brief conversation. Regardless of whether the subject is at a distance, practitioners may focus their attention on the intended subject, as they then test the surrogate in their presence with the help of their EMT Long Form. Whether performed locally or nonlocally, the results are consistently remarkable.

In either case, if a subject's given organ reveals deficient energy, the practitioner will want to stimulate it by circling their dominant

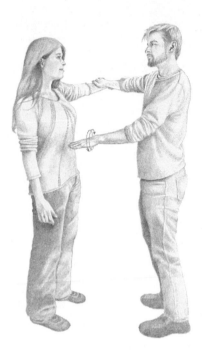

FIGURE 5.6   *Wenchiech'u*

hand in counterclockwise motions to add much-needed energy. If the subject indicates excess energy, the practitioner should cool the subject down by motioning their hand in a clockwise direction. Always remember that the subject is the clock facing outward. This means that counterclockwise (strengthening energy) would circle to their right. Clockwise (draining energy) would circle to their left (see Figure 5.6). It is important to clarify that clockwise is yang and counterclockwise is yin. However, due to the fact that these are fluid and not static forces, each is always transitioning into the opposite. So clockwise is yang, which produces yin energy. Counterclockwise is yin, which produces yang energy. In this way, clockwise spirals release excess energy and counterclockwise spirals add to or rebalance deficient energy.

I am often asked questions like "What if I accidentally spin the spirals in the wrong direction, will I harm the subject?" No, you will not. Once the practitioner sets their intention, any spirals that may be accidentally transmitted in the wrong direction will automatically be corrected by the wave of intention. As already stated, willpower and concentration are the most important variables because they generate an intense wave of intention.

PAIN POINT WENCHIECH'U

In the event that you're finding it difficult to muddle through all the confusion of energy diagnostics and point-and-zone location, you always have the option of simply aiming your Wenchiech'u treatment at what I call the pain point—that is, wherever it hurts. Wenchiech'u is a single-action protocol, so there is no need to worry about where the excesses or deficiencies are, and no need to perform organ balancing. It's strictly about making pain stop where it's manifesting, not necessarily where it's rooted. For example, if your subject has an inflammatory headache, you'll want to circle your dominant hand counterclockwise around their head. Ask them exactly where the root of their pain is and try your best to zero right in on the focal point of their disharmony. This enables you to engage your healing intentions right away.

I am often asked how long it takes to perform a Wenchiech'u treatment and how long it generally lasts. Treatments should last no longer than two minutes and generally last for three weeks, depending on the acuteness of the subject's condition or disease. Acute conditions such as influenza viruses typically require daily boosting. Chronic conditions and diseases, even if severe, require less boosting and are generally fine to boost at three-week intervals. You can never do harm by overboosting! Regardless of human error, no wrong can come of Wenchiech'u. All human error and ill intention is automatically canceled out.

THE WENCHIECH'U LONGEVITY EXERCISE

The ancient Chinese often emphasized the importance of longevity as a means to immortality. They understood that your true "self" is rooted in spirit, and spirit is immortal. Therefore, immortality is something that cannot be attained, but rather, is only realized. This is true immortality. Living a full, abundant life for 120 years as nature intended us to allows us sufficient time to cultivate true spiritual wisdom. To further enable us to cultivate this age-old wisdom, they formulated eight secrets of longevity.

Eight Secrets of Longevity

1. Abolish self-limitation.
2. Hear your inner nature.
3. Eat purely.
4. Exercise your body routinely.
5. Maintain a strong positive attitude.
6. Maintain regular spiritual practice.
7. Avoid addiction.
8. The last secret is one that only you can discover within.

Here in the modern West, the concept of longevity is more about staving off untimely death and living as healthful for as possible for a long lifetime. As we've discussed, in recent years, Western science has made some remarkable discoveries regarding longevity and how to lengthen the telomeres, which protect our DNA from "fraying" each time our cells divide. Science is continuing to discover that diet, lifestyle, and stress management all contribute to telomere protection and repair. It won't come as a surprise to anyone who has ever experimented with any of these things, that proper diet, certain nutritional supplements, regular exercise, meditation, and Qigong have all been found to repair and extend lon-

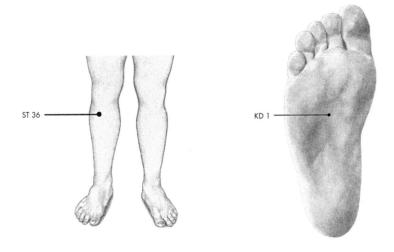

ST 36

KD 1

FIGURE 5.7   *The Longevity Points*

gevity. Wenchiech'u is one form of Qigong that can, if practiced properly, support longevity.

The previous chapter discussed longevity diagnosis. Here we will reveal EMT techniques for balancing body energy to stimulate telomere activity and enhance its longevity powers. Practitioner and subject should already have completed the diagnostic portion of this exercise and should therefore already be interfaced and tuned. Assuming that the subject was found to have a deficient longevity point (ST 36 or KD 1), they are in need of Wenchiech'u stimulation. Therefore, the practitioner's intention should be to spin highly charged, compressed, counterclockwise energy directly at the subject's deficient longevity point. This will require a good minute and a half of spinning the energy. It is also very important to note that advanced practitioners may use the Grasping the Ch'i method to diagnose their own longevity points. They might also, in effect, balance themselves by spinning the Wenchiech'u energy counterclockwise at their own deficient longevity points.

Weaving and fluttering the ch'i will also enhance the longevity points. Each of these techniques is an excellent vehicle for directing the healing power of ch'i. As long as the practitioner's mind remains focused and their intention wave has been generated, the ch'i will effectively transmit where it is intended to go.

CHAPTER 6

WHOLE HEALTH NUTRITIONAL BALANCING: FOOD AS MEDICINE

FOOD IS MEDICINE!

I recently viewed a superb program on PBS that reexamined the theories about our split from the apes. The show was based on the work of paleontologists Martin Pickford and Brigitte Senut from the Collège de France. In the Tugen Hills of Kenya, the two scientists recently unearthed what they have named *Orrorin tugenensis*—a six-million-year-old hominid and, some experts believe, the oldest ancestor we have.

As I watched in amazement, I couldn't help but wonder how *Orrorin tugenensis* lived. I thought, "Did they somehow manage to prosper in the face of hardship? And how did they heal themselves when they were sick and wounded? What did they eat?" These ancient ancestors contain the blueprint for our biochemical hardwiring. What lessons about life, survival, food, and natural medicine might we learn from them?

Biological life has been evolving on this planet for more than three billion years. The first primates are said to have roamed the earth as far back as 65000000 BC. Their earliest diet was said to have consisted of insects. It wasn't until approximately 50000000 BC that our primate predecessors began eating fruits and vegetables. Until the work of Pickford and Senut forces anthropology to reconsider, the appearance of the first true humans, *Homo habilis* ("handy man"), is believed to be around 2300000 BC. These hunter-gatherers subsisted on a diet that was 60 to 70 percent fruits and vegetables, and only about 30 to 40 percent flesh. For more than two million years and twenty civilizations, our earliest ancestors were forced to become master adaptors in order to survive.

Throughout their evolution, our ancestors had no choice but to develop systems of eating and healing, utilizing whatever natural resources were available to them. Limited by the dictates of season, climate, weather, and indigenous availability, they managed to prosper, grow, and heal masterfully. The earliest dawning of modern civilization, some 4,000 to 5,000 years ago, saw the most antiquated systems of organized recorded medicine. Ancient Chinese, Ayurvedic, Babylonian, Egyptian, Greek, Native American, Persian, and Roman systems of natural medicine all looked first to food and herbs to invoke cure.

Food was the first medicine. As far back as 4,000 years ago, the Egyptians used asparagus as a diuretic. The Maya used papaya fruit to aid digestion. The ancient Menominee tribe of North America used the seeds of pumpkin to expel worms. Both the Greeks and Romans used carrot seeds to stimulate menstruation and relieve urinary retention. The Egyptians, Romans, Greeks, Hindus, and Mesopotamians employed more than 500 "vegetable drugs," powerful druglike agents from foods and herbs. Pliny the Elder, a Roman naturalist and author of a massive encyclopedia of the natural world, taught that cabbage cured eighty-seven diseases, and onions cured twenty-eight. The Romans believe that lentils balanced mood.

They also used grapes in their medicinal preparations for enemas, as well as for skin and breathing problems. History is rife with accounts of food cures that changed the fate of mankind.

Scurvy, once a dreaded medical condition of the skin and gums resulting from vitamin C deficiency, was cured by common foods. In 1753, Scottish surgeon James Lind of the British Royal Navy was the first to document the scurvy-healing properties of citrus fruits, such as lemons and limes.

Rickets, a disease marked by a softening of the bones, is the result of vitamin D deficiency. The ancient Chinese were said to have cured this disease centuries ago with the use of fish oils.

Pernicious anemia—a progressive, degenerative disease of the nervous system that can lead to severe neurological symptoms such as those associated with MS and Parkinson's disease—is caused by vitamin B_{12} deficiency. It was considered fatal until 1926 when Nobel Prize–winning researcher George H. Whipple discovered that with the help of dietary raw liver, the disease was no longer fatal.

Nearly seventy years ago, Weston A. Price, a Cleveland dentist and researcher, set out to study the natural diets of civilizations the world over. He was convinced that degenerative conditions such as rampant tooth decay, arthritis, osteoporosis, diabetes, and chronic fatigue were the direct result of denatured, processed foods (foods with processed sugars, white flours, rancid and chemically altered oils and fats). Especially disturbed by the frequent infections, allergies, asthma, and behavioral problems among the many children he treated, Dr. Price was inspired to make a difference. He traveled to many isolated corners of the globe to study the health, physical development, and diets of those inhabitants who had no previous contact with modern civilization. His research took him to remote Swiss villages; isolated Scottish islands; the Florida Everglades; northernmost Eskimo fishing villages; and indigenous communities in Australia, New Zealand, Peru, Africa, and the Amazon. In every region he traveled to, he found villages and tribes where the natives commonly exhibited what Dr. Price called "natural physical perfection." In addition, they exhibited an almost complete absence of disease.

Interesting to note, however, was the stark contrast in health, structure, and development among these peoples after missionaries had changed their native diets to modern diets. Dr. Price found that it took no more than one generation on processed, denatured foods to seriously degrade their overall health and well-being.

The natural diets of all these people were varied, but the foods that Dr. Price summarized as the most superior for optimal health were fish, organ meats, whole grains, vegetables, fruits, clabbered milks (yogurt), and tubers. Price's research clearly demonstrates that food has been our medicine since the beginning of time.

BACK TO THE FUTURE

With the aid of anthropological research, we are once again beginning to learn what our ancestors innately knew about the medicinal power of food. Like their ancestors, approximately 75 percent of the world's population continues to rely on food as medicine. More than 25 percent of our prescriptive drugs today are derived from common foods, plants, shrubs, and herbs.

Many astounding food studies are now setting the stage for a future that will most certainly spotlight food as *the* preeminent medicine.

Studies have confirmed that foods act as anticoagulants, antidepressants, antiulcerants, antithrombotics, analgesics, tranquilizers, sedatives, cholesterol reducers, cancer fighters, natural chemotherapy agents, preventatives, hormone regulators, fertility agents, laxatives, antidiarrheal agents, immune stimulators, biological response modifiers, antihypertensives, diuretics, decongestants, antibiotics, antiviral agents, antinausea agents, cough suppressants, blood vessel dilators, and bronchial dilators.

Included in recent groundbreaking "food is medicine" research are studies that have confirmed that fish oil, garlic, walnuts, flax-seeds, olive oil, red wine, oat bran, onions, avocados, grapes, green vegetables, and hot peppers help to reverse heart disease by triggering anti-inflammatory hormones.

Garlic, onions, grapes, soy, walnuts, flaxseeds, pumpkin seeds, and fatty fish have been proven to prevent blood clots, while citrus, berries, tomatoes, cabbage, carrots, scallions, broccoli, celery, green peppers, cucumbers, dark lettuce, beans, tea, fish oils, and whole grains help prevent cancer. Bananas, beans, cabbage, licorice, cayenne pepper, and hot chili peppers help to heal ulcers, while celery, garlic, and potassium-rich fruits such as figs, dates, raisins, bananas, and avocados help to lower blood pressure. Let's take a closer look at the medicinal properties of food from a current, scientific perspective.

THE MEDICINAL PROPERTIES OF FOOD (PHYTOCHEMICALS)

Phytochemicals are nutrients found in plant-based foods. They have existed since the beginning of plant life on Earth, and our ancient ancestors were the first to observe their many potential healing properties. Today, following decades of research, more than 4,000 phytochemicals have been identified, and approximately 100 have been intensively studied for their medicinal properties. Some phytochemicals commonly found in fruits, vegetables, whole grains, and herbs are extremely rich in powerful medicinal properties that can actually help prevent—and even cure—disease.

Researchers have identified three key ways that phytochemicals help boost human immunity. Their powerful antioxidants help neutralize disease-causing free radicals. They also help eliminate toxic wastes by manipulating phase 1 and phase 2 enzymes, and regulate disease-causing hormones. Some important categories of phytochemicals include:

1. *Carotenoids*—Found in carrots, tomatoes, broccoli, peppers, and cantaloupe. They help prevent stomach, prostate, lung, and colon cancer as well as lower the risk of heart disease. In addition they reduce the incidence of age-related macular degeneration and cataracts.

2. *Allylic sulfides*—Found in garlic, onions, scallions, and leeks. They raise good cholesterol, lower bad fats, and stimulate immune enzymes that antagonize tumor development.

3. *Phenolic compounds*—Found in most vegetables, whole grains, green and black teas, and fruits. They mobilize enzymes that inhibit cancers of the bladder, breast, colon, liver, blood, pancreas, skin, and stomach.

4. *Isoflavones*—Found in beans and legumes (soy). They lower toxic estrogen levels and antagonize certain cancers, as well as reduce risks for hot flashes and osteoporosis.

5. *Saponins*—Found in asparagus, spinach, tomatoes, soy, and beans. They prevent heart disease and certain cancers, and remove dangerous cholesterol from the body.

6. *Flavonoids*—Found in citrus, grapes, berries, green leafy vegetables, and onions. They help inhibit cancers of the breast, lung, and stomach. They also help reverse atherosclerosis, antagonize toxic hormones, and fortify collagen.

7. *Monoterpenes*—Found in cherries and citrus. They produce enzymes that block breast, pancreatic, lung, skin, and stomach cancer–causing compounds. They also reduce arterial plaque formation.

This brief mention doesn't do justice to the real phytochemical story. Phytochemical studies are ongoing, as scientific research is increasingly turning to food as a new source of medicine. At this point, researchers have barely uncovered the tip of the iceberg concerning the potential healing powers of food. What our ancestors learned empirically, we are learning scientifically. Different methods that result in the same discovery—food is medicine.

SOME PERSONAL STORIES

I recently worked with a thirty-five-year-old man who suffered from high blood pressure, elevated cholesterol, and type 2 diabetes. His HMO had put him on a high-starch diet and his doctors had prescribed a number of medications. In spite of those treatment protocols, all of his conditions continued to worsen. The only suggestion his doctors could offer was to increase his medications. That's when he decided to pay me a visit.

I immediately took him off the high-starch diet and placed him on a Whole Health nutrition plan with a high-protein, low-starch carbohydrate diet. I've found that high-starch diets tend to increase the need for insulin, which many diabetics aren't able to sufficiently produce. Higher protein intake increases the production of the hormone glucagon, which takes the pressure off the pancreas by requiring less insulin.

Next, following his Whole Health EMT evaluation, I put him on megadoses of chromium (a mineral supplement) to help balance out his blood sugar, vitamin B_3 and Indian gooseberry to lower his cholesterol, and pycnogenol (French maritime pine bark) and bonita fish peptide to lower his blood pressure.

He was a disciplined patient who followed his program as well as anybody I have ever worked with. After only three months, he went back to his doctor for a checkup. His cholesterol had dropped from 260 to 170, his blood sugars had completely normalized (well below the renal threshold), and his blood pressure was perfect!

When he told his doctor that he had accomplished all of this by following a natural regime of diet and supplements, his doctor proceeded to scold him.

Nonetheless, I continue to see him for follow-up visits, and he remains symptom free and off all medications. His food is now his medicine.

When it comes to "food as medicine," there's yet another side to the story. A thirty-five-year-old man, a veteran of the First Gulf War, recently came to see me with a long list of troubling symptoms. For two years, he had been experiencing chronic stomach cramps, severe gas, nausea, diarrhea, an increased urge to urinate, drooling, sweating, headaches, dizziness, eye tearing, blurred vision, a runny nose, shortness of breath, acid reflux, tingling of the extremities (fingers, toes, arms, and legs), muscle twitching, cramping, and weakness.

At first glance, he looked like a man in good health because he was physically fit, had perfect posture, a very balanced temperament, and appeared to be very emotionally and mentally stable. After recording his history, I was baffled by the wide range of his symptoms until he told me the rest of his story.

He explained that while serving in the Persian Gulf, he and a number of his fellow soldiers were forced by the U.S. military, against their will, to take a number of toxic agents. He explained to me that they were given oral doses of pyridostigmine bromide. This drug is also known under the trade names Mestinon and Regonol, and it is intended to combat the effects of drug toxicity. The problem is that it has been implicated as a causal factor in Gulf War syndrome because of its known side effects—nausea, vomiting, diarrhea, cramps, and tearing.

He told me that they were also forced to take 30 mg doses of anthrax bacteria orally every eight hours. Anthrax—*Bacillus anthracis*—is an acute, rapidly developing bacterial infection of the skin, lungs, and intestinal tract. According to investigative reporter Gary Matsumoto, the army used an unlicensed, experimental anthrax vaccine that contained squalene, a dangerous, oil-based adjuvant. Adjuvants like squalene tend to intensify the effects of whatever else is contained in vaccines. Squalene has been shown to cause permanent organ damage and irreversible autoimmune disease in animal trials.

The U.S. Army contends that they were advised to administer such treatments for the purpose of building up resistance in the event of combat exposures.

I immediately began his EMT and food energy testing. I discovered extensive energy weakness in his nervous system, caused by an exposure to neurotoxins. It was as if he had a neurodegenerative disease. Not surprisingly, I also discovered that he had a number of severe food allergies. His immune system was clearly compromised from the toxic exposures, and his diet was obstructing his body's efforts to throw off the toxins.

We completed his Whole Health energy diagnosis and put together a comprehensive program. I asked him to strictly avoid all his food allergens, as well as all fermented foods, and to take neurological-supporting and immune-supporting supplements— methyl B_{12} (5,000 mcg) and propolis (2,000 mg). I also recommended that he take a homeopathic detoxification medicine called Drugtox from Molecular Biologics—ten drops under the tongue twice a day, to help remove elements of the pyridostigmine bromide he'd been given in the army.

I further recommended microdoses of anthricinum—homeopathic anthrax bacteria. Like using snake venom antidote, homeopathy is a safe way to antidote toxic exposures. These once-toxic substances are formulated into dilutions beyond any material trace, on the principle that there is energy remaining within the existing molecules. By exposing a subject to an extremely diluted homeopathic medicine that was once a toxin, you can safely stimulate their immunity to detoxify it from their system.

I am pleased to report that after six months of our working together, he is symptom free. He tells me that he feels as though he's gotten his life back together at last. Here's the key—I believe that his avoidance of food allergens and fermented foods such as vinegars, yeasted breads, processed sugars, and marinated foods was the main reason for his recovery. Food allergens obstruct the liver and large intestines, and fermented foods produce ammonia and acetic, lactic, pyruvic, and carbonic acids in the body, making it virtually impossible for the body to naturally detoxify endotoxic poisons.

His is a classic case of "food as medicine" from the "addition through subtraction" perspective. The Whole Health philosophy emphasizes that the first guideline for food as medicine is "It's not just about what you add—it's also about what you subtract!"

SUBTRACT TOXIC FOOD

The first and most basic step in Whole Health Healing is to subtract toxic food from the diet. When it comes to health care problem solving, ours is a culture that tends to add, not subtract. To heal you and rid you of your symptoms and maladies, the present approach offers to add special diets, detoxification plans, vitamins, herbal remedies, medications, and the like. This approach to health care is largely the result of "problem-solution" programming. "You've got a problem—we'll sell you the solution." This is also a very disempowering approach, as it makes the patient more codependent on the solution, and they cannot supply the solution themselves. Take inflammation, for example. Seventy-two percent of all inflammatory disease is the result of poor diet. Inflammatory diseases, like some cancers, heart disease, lupus, and rheumatoid arthritis, come about because of elevated COX-2 hormones, which are the result of elevated arachidonic fatty acid, which comes about from overconsumption of red meat, dairy, egg yolks, peanuts, and sugar. Instead of empowering patients by teaching them to eat fewer inflammatory foods, the present health care system opts to prescribe them steroids. The side effects of the steroids often cause serious side effects, especially with long-term use, and they further send the patient's body a message to turn off their innate anti-inflammatory chemistry.

Remember, the Whole Health approach is the result of more than thirty years and 60,000 consultations. It has been proven to be effective time and time again. This section on subtracting toxic foods isn't intended to take all of the fun out of life! The intention is rather to offer an effective nutritional protocol for those interested in healing chronic or acute health conditions. If it seems overwhelmingly restrictive, Whole Health advises you to consider taking its twenty-one-day challenge. Just follow the plan for twenty-one days and reevaluate. Your mind and body will work it out from there. The more common strategy recommended by Whole Health is to abide by its 85 percent law. That is, you follow the plan strictly during the week (this is the 85 percent) and take two meals off (within reason) on weekends (this is the 15 percent). Most notice the distinct contrast between how great they feel by Thursday and Friday and how poorly they feel on Sunday night. Again, your mind and body will work it out.

When it comes to toxic food subtraction, the first rule of thumb is to know exactly what you want from your food. Then you will know precisely what you're going to get. You must consciously choose the experience you want to get from your food—neutral, medicinal, or toxic. Whole Health recognizes three categories of toxic food: junk food, fermented food, and inflammatory food. The first step to eliminating toxic food is to subtract junk food.

Junk Food Subtraction List

Processed sugars	Pies
Fried foods	Cookies
White flour	Ice cream
White rice	Fast food
Cakes	Juices

Soft drinks	Condiments
Pizza	Gravies
Hot dogs	Sour cream
Cold cuts	Alcohol
Creamed soups	

Then there's the issue of additives. If you can't pronounce the chemical ingredients in your foods, don't risk them! To get the full medicinal value, make the commitment to consistently consume only truly organic food. The Organic Foods Production Act assures the consumer that any food product with a "100 percent Organic" label is truly organic. Products labeled "Organic" must be at least 95 percent organic.

The second type of toxic food to subtract on the Whole Health plan is fermented food. There is a great deal of confusion about fermented food. Many people are quick to point out theories that suggest that fermentation has a medicinal value. For example, they may make mention of the many immune-enhancing studies of medicinal fungi, such as kombucha. Still others may point to the fact that fermented soy has been shown to neutralize phytic acid, which is detrimental to nutrient absorption. Some would be quick to point out that sauerkraut produces probiotic benefits that support intestinal flora.

Whole Health posits that there are inconsistencies with fermentation, and not all human chemistries have the capability to safely assimilate it. It comes down to a matter of risk and reward. The rewards are potentially great, but so are the risks. For those who can't effectively process fermentation, their bodies may produce toxins, such as acetic acid, lactic acid, pyruvic acid, carbonic acid, and ammonia. With fermentation, there is simply no middle ground. You'd better get it right! In the words of two-time Nobel Prize winner Dr. Otto Warburg: "The prime cause of cancer is the replacement of the respiration of oxygen in normal body cells with the fermentation of sugar."

Fermented Food Subtraction List

Yeasted breads	Beer
Mushrooms	Wine
Truffles	Champagne
Vinegars	Fermented soy (miso, tempeh,
Nuts	tamari)
Seeds	Aged cheeses (blue, Limburger,
Melons	cheddar, Parmesan, Asiago)

The third and final toxic food avoidance category is inflammatory food. The topic of inflammation has changed dramatically over the past twenty-five years. Not too long ago, the world thought of inflammation as a bad case of tennis elbow. Following the 1930 discovery of eicosanoid molecules as a component of semen by gynecologist Raphael Kurzrok and pharmacologist Charles Leib, our understanding of inflammation began to change and expand.

Today we know that eicosanoids (signaling molecules), often referred to as "local" hormones, are where inflammation and anti-inflammation patterns begin in the human body. Eicosanoids are called signaling molecules because they send communication commands to cells, molecules, and hormones. In relaying these commands, they initiate the body's production of inflammatory and anti-inflammatory mechanisms. When you consider that experts now believe that 72 percent of all disease is the result of inflammatory programming, this is a very important aspect of biochemistry. Now for the clincher—fats trigger both the inflammatory and anti-inflammatory systems. The fat that triggers inflammation is arachidonic acid. Where do we get inflammatory arachidonic fatty acid? We get it from foods. Therefore, foods trigger the inflammation responsible for 72 percent of all disease. The inflammatory process is global in the human body, affecting virtually every anatomical system. Elevated levels of arachidonic acid can result in heart disease (blood clots), cancer, lupus, rheumatoid arthritis, migraine headaches, and numerous other ailments. The subtraction of inflammatory foods represents a significant factor in the three decades of success of the Whole Health System.

Inflammatory Food Subtraction List

Food allergens

Red meats

Dairy products

Egg yolks

Nuts (especially peanuts)

Nori

Seaweed

Tilapia

Catfish

Duck

Fried foods

Yellowtail (Japanese
  amberjack)

Most vegetable oils (except for
  olive and flaxseed oils)

Processed sugars and starches

FOOD ALLERGY/INTOLERANCE SUBTRACTION

I recently worked with a fourteen-year-old boy with severe malabsorption. His digestion was so severely impaired, he was unable to digest any fats, 75 percent of his carbohydrates, and more than 60 percent of his proteins. The boy's health became further jeopardized due to the buildup of high levels of fungal bacteria in his gut, resulting from malabsorption of starches and sugars.

At their wits' end, his parents took him to the gastroenterology department at one of the more well-known Boston hospitals. Due to the fact that he was losing a great deal of weight, the gastroenterology department referred the family to one of the hospital's registered dieticians. The dietician proceeded to recommend that the boy commence a steady diet of BOOST brand milk shakes and muffins to help him gain weight. The problem is, the boy was severely allergic to dairy and wheat, but because the gastroenterology department didn't believe in the food allergy testing protocol, and lacked education in food science, the family was ordered to keep the boy on the milk shakes and muffins. He continued to complain of severe gastric pain from the diet. When his parents requested a healthier dietary plan for their son, the gastroenterologist threatened to report the parents to the state Department of Social Services to have the child removed from the home on the grounds of parental neglect if they failed to maintain the diet.

I saw the boy in my office, EMT tested him for food allergies, designed a meal plan from the list of foods that passed, and within six weeks he was clear of his condition.

ACID/ALKALINE BALANCE

Inflammatory foods are problematic for more than one reason. One very important problem generated by inflammation is acidosis. Acid robs cells of oxygen, while alkalinity donates oxygen to cells. Our bodies and minds move through cyclical rhythms triggered by light, temperature, and diet. Among our many cycles are a seven-day and a twenty-eight-day biorhythm cycle. We also have a twenty-four-hour metabolic cycle, during which certain hours are favored for specific body functions. For example, digestion is best suited between the hours of 7:00 a.m. and 3:00 p.m., while tissue repair takes place between the hours of 3:00 p.m. and 11:00 p.m. The third metabolic cycle, when the body detoxifies itself, occurs between 11:00 p.m. and 7:00 a.m. One of the key cornerstones for supporting these metabolic cycles is maintaining a stable dietary pH.

Most fruits and vegetables are alkaline, while animal foods, most grains, nuts, seeds, and processed foods are acidic. Earlier I quoted Dr. Otto Warburg, who underscored the importance of maintaining alkalinity by reminding us that the primary cause of cancer is the fermentation of sugar. Fermentation and sugar generate acid-producing systems, which initiate the degeneration of healthy cells. Whole Health recommends testing the urine on occasion with pHydrion 0.067 calibrated urine strips. Test the morning's urine first. These strips reflect a pH range between 5.0 and 8.0. Optimal balance is reflected in a first morning's urine between 6.4 and 6.8. If acidic (below 6.4), increase vegetable, fruit, and pure water consumption and take ¼ teaspoon of baking soda in water before bed at night. If levels don't correct within three weeks, add two tablespoons of liquid chlorophyll in six ounces of water, three times daily. Both the baking soda and chlorophyll doses may be doubled if necessary. Continue testing urine.

Note: those with high blood pressure should use liquid chlorophyll instead of baking soda. Take 1 tablespoon mixed with a few ounces of water—three times daily.

SUBTRACTING FOOD ALLERGENS
AND INTOLERANCES

Many of my patients struggle with the notion that they are as sensitive to foods as they are, and refuse to believe it. A woman I recently saw had just returned from a cruise with friends. As she explained it, her friends ate everything from soup to nuts. She, on the other hand, cut just a few minor corners, only to get pounded with severe inflammatory symptoms. She was distraught, to say the least.

I explained to her that each and every one of us fits into one of two categories. I categorize one group as acute/chronic types and the other as chronic/acute types. I wanted her to understand that she needn't feel so all alone with her food problem. While she may be acutely sensitive to foods, by adhering to her anti-inflammatory, hypoallergenic diet, her overall health would improve dramatically— at the chronic level—over time. On the other hand, her friends on the cruise who ate virtually everything in sight may be more tolerant at the acute level, but they are more likely to suffer from chronic disease over the course of time. The state of our dietary practices in America today is becoming an increasingly serious problem.

Over the past three decades, there has been growing interest in food intolerances and food allergies. It's estimated that as many as 90 million Americans suffer from either genetic food intolerances or food allergies of some kind. Food intolerances are responses that occur when something in a given food irritates a person's digestive system. Symptoms may include rash, hives, nausea, diarrhea, itchy skin, shortness of breath, chest pain, swelling of bronchial passageways, and anaphylaxis.

Food allergies are an immune reaction. They occur when the body's autoimmune intelligence activates in defensive response to a food by producing antibodies to the food, as if the food were an invading pathogen. Allergic food reactions are varied, and may include stomach pains, hives, headaches, asthma, bronchial congestion, muscle and joint aches, nausea—and even irrational, "neurotic" emotional and mental behavior. The most common allergens are milk and dairy products, wheat, corn, shellfish, citrus, legumes (including peas, beans, soy products, and inflammatory nuts such as peanuts), eggs, and "nightshade" vegetables or fruits such as tomatoes, eggplant, peppers, and cabbages.

To clinically confirm a food allergy, diagnosis requires either a radioallergosorbent skin test (RAST), where the skin is scratched and exposed to food extracts to observe antibody reactions, or immunoglobulin blood tests, in which blood platelets are exposed to food extracts so that they will display either positive or negative aggregation response.

When you understand the why and how of food allergies and intolerances, it's easy to see why they are so common. If, for twenty-five of the past thirty generations, a family gene pool was not exposed to dairy products, and therefore lacked specialized enzymes capable of digesting milk, there would be a strong probability for dairy allergies.

In his noted article "The Significance of Mutation in Preventive Dentistry," Hal Huggins, D.D.S., wrote of "an ancestral dietary concept, which is based upon the hypothesis that a species lives and eats the foods in one area for 1,000 years or more, and becomes adapted to the foods in that area. If a species moves to a new habitat, it comes in contact with new foods that require different intestinal bacteria to digest them, and modifications must be made. The species may need another 1,000 years to adapt to the new diet." (*Let's Live*, March 1989, p. 68.)

Digestion is highly specialized, substantially increasing the likelihood of food intolerances wherever there exists an overexpanded variety, abundance, and/or volume of food.

Just think, there are 75 trillion cells in our bodies, with more than 1,000 enzymes (many of which are digestive) at work in each cell. Most enzymes participate in only one chemical reaction upon a single substance, although some do act upon compounds. There are, on average, more than 50,000 digestive enzymes in the body, some specifically for protein digestion (proteases), some for fat digestion (lipases), and some for carbohydrate digestion (amylases). A single cell contains thousands of enzymes for thousands of different specialized actions. At the same time, each food, according to its classification, requires separate enzymes and enzyme compounds to perform various functions in the digestive process. Each food falls within a specific pH (acid/alkaline) range that dictates the efficiency with which each enzyme performs its work, just as each enzyme performs optimally at a specific pH.

The less work required of our digestive systems, the more efficient the digestion. The more overworked a digestive system, as is often the case today, the more nondigestive toxic residues build up in the body. This buildup requires immune antibodies to neutralize their subsequent pathogenic presence.

As long as allergens are being ingested, the immune system must continually engage in reaction to them. This constant preoccupation with food-related toxins forces the immune defense system to become distracted from its other important functions, such as protection from invasive bacteria and viruses, as well as immune antibody and DNA repair.

Accumulated toxicity from food allergens also forms degenerative concentrations of protein putrefaction and starch fermentation in the colon, both of which interfere with our protective microfloral (bacterial) synthesis. The predominant bacteria in the colon, *Escherichia coli*, are employed to release such gases as methane, carbon dioxide, hydrogen, lactic and acetic acid, as well as such toxic gases as indole and phenol. These protective *E. coli* bacteria are also responsible for the microbial synthesis of the vitamins and minerals responsible for our body's daily maintenance functions. I believe that these toxic accumulations in the colon from food intolerances are a major cause of Americans' weakened immunities.

Many current health care practitioners believe that food allergies, despite the fact that they are one of the most misunderstood and undiagnosed issues, remain one of the truly primary causes of the present health care crisis. As the body, mind, and spirit are continually bombarded with the stressful tasks of adapting to modern life, there is a breakdown in digestion. Stress often predetermines digestive efficiency, and thus, food tolerance. As this breakdown spreads its inflammatory influence to other body systems, it may well begin to paint a more systemic picture of immunosuppression.

I have found that blood and skin tests alone are not reliable enough in determining food intolerances and allergies. I have consistently observed thousands of patients who have been clinically tested and cleared, but continue to exhibit severe symptoms from food intolerances and allergies, and I believe this to be one of the most important, yet nebulous, areas of health care.

I have noted that no two people react the same to any one allergen. For example, one person exposed to a dairy allergen might exhibit migraine headaches while another exhibits bronchial congestion. Furthermore, a person might be exposed to a food one day and show no reaction, while as many as five days later a severe latent reaction might occur. To further complicate matters, the symptoms might be as elusive as a slight mood shift, or mental "fog."

An array of self-help diet books instruct their readers about "rotation diets," which are designed to allow the digestive tract time to clear itself before a certain food is eaten again. For example, if I were to eat apples on Monday, then I would abstain from apples for the next three days and eat apples again on Friday. There are many variations on this theme, with each advocate adding a personal theory and a change here and there. Nonetheless, the basis for rotation remains the same—simplifying the digestive workload.

Just as with blood and skin tests, the flaw in rotation diets is that they are either too general or they fail to consistently address subtle energetic human responses (thoughts and emotions) to potential allergens. We are composed of energy, which makes up 99.999 percent of our matter. The very innermost core from which our entire being emanates is composed of energy. Whole Health asserts that the secret to a more accurate diagnostic testing lies in the sixth-sensory potential of our unconscious mind, and the ever-changing field of energy it generates.

FOOD ENERGY

When it comes to material diagnostics, the Western world remains at the forefront. We've developed remarkable technologies that enable physicians to analyze the status of one's health via the mediums of blood, saliva, urine, and DNA. The Western world has clearly devoted itself to a material bias, but as the new millennium unfolds, there is a growing interest in the potentials and applications of energy-healing systems.

When I began developing the Whole Health system more than thirty years ago, I had no more than an innate knowing about self, world, and universe as conjoined parts of one unified energy field. And while my first visions of food as medicine were simply attuned to concepts of clean, healthy, and organic eating, I had no real technical understanding of how the energy of food could affect the energy of human beings. Like the rest of my culture, I believed that "food as medicine" was all about good nutrition, and that good nutrition was strictly about material nutrients. Yet somehow I also felt that there was much more to it all.

As I began my work, I immediately noticed that thoughts, emotions, climate, weather, lifestyle, relationships, and dreams all had a way of exerting a profound effect on all of the people I was counseling.

I will never forget a young woman who came to see me who was constantly sick with colds and flu, and allergic to virtually everything she was surrounded by. I recommended a healthier diet and some natural vitamins, to no avail. Then one fateful day, toward the end of an office visit, she happened to mention that she and her husband were not getting along. She began to open up to me, explaining that he was a verbally abusive, imperative type and that she was very intimidated by him. I simply shared some uplifting words of encouragement and reminded her, "We are all only as powerful as our willingness to be so, and as deserving as our willingness to affirm." I didn't see her for many months. I thought that perhaps I'd overstepped my boundaries. Then, many months later, she came knocking on my door. I barely recognized her! She looked transformed. No longer immunosuppressed, and no longer having allergic reactions, she was absolutely radiant. She proceeded to tell me that she had been profoundly moved by our earlier conversation and that it inspired her to find the strength to demand that her husband leave the house. He did so—and she moved on to lead a much happier, fuller, healthier life.

I felt awakened to the power of subtle human energy. This experience made me acutely aware of the fact that subtle energies from within us make all the difference in the realms of our material human health. All the health food and vitamins in the world couldn't do for her what only her mind could. Her experience represents all of us. She made it clear to me that she and you and I have not yet been fully accounted for within the present health care system. She couldn't be doctored. She had to be healed. What she had couldn't be tested in her blood, saliva, urine, or DNA.

As the years went on, her face was accompanied by thousands of other faces. Someone has to stretch the present limitations, I remember thinking. We can't continue to simply run material tests and give out material medicines to all these people. They are comprised of vital energies that require attention as well.

RAW VERSUS COOKED FOOD

The question of raw versus cooked food can only be answered through personalization. Whole Health is a system that ascribes to energetic individuality. We are comprised of a myriad of subtle energies and we are all very different and ever changing. Whole Health therefore suggests that the question of raw versus cooked food be individually tested and retested each season. As the seasons change, we change. Simply use the EMT pass/fail testing technique. Hold up your partner's arm and test their strength response when calling out the terms: *cold/raw food* and *warm/cooked food*. You will instantly resolve the great debate!

THE WHOLE HEALTH WEIGHT LOSS PLAN

For those interested, here's a sample Whole Health meal plan designed for general weight loss.

	PROTEIN	VEGETABLES/FRUIT	HIGH-STARCH CARBS
BREAKFAST	4 egg whites or 3 organic poultry links	6 ounces	None
A.M. SNACK	None	1 fruit	None
LUNCH	6 ounces lean poultry, fish, or beans	6 ounces (If having a salad, dress with 2 tablespoons of olive oil and lemon—avoid vinegar.)	None
P.M. SNACK	None	1/3 ripe avocado or 2 tablespoons organic soy nut butter	8–10 organic plain rice crackers
DINNER	6 ounces lean poultry, fish, or beans	6 ounces	6 ounces (brown rice, brown rice pasta, or 1 white or sweet potato)
EVENING SNACK	None	None	None

A NOTE ABOUT EMOTIONAL EATING DISORDERS

It is estimated that eight million Americans have eating disorders of one kind or another. Seven million are said to be women. I recently saw a woman who said, "I have an eating disorder." She said it in such an affirming way, she seemed to link the condition with her identity. I reminded her that she wasn't an eating disorder, but rather she was a sensitive human being with a potentially broken heart. Some overeat the pain away with food. Some stop eating, as they are fearful of eating too much, gaining weight, and risking rejection because of being unattractive. I have often explained to my patients that many of us who are overwhelmed with heartache suffer from the continued subconscious recall of our emotional pain. These painful images and feelings continue to revisit our nervous system. Substances that appear to offer immediate gratification (like foods) then become our chosen distraction. They offer no long-term help. They typically only leave us with continued suffering and accompanying health problems.

I suggest to my patients that they distill the issue down to a "feed or feel" proposition. They can either continue to try in desperation to feed the pain back down, or they can feel the pain out. I suggest that they begin looking at their pain as mere energy. Consciously deemphasize all stigmas and associations. Try to release the memories of the people, places, and things involved with your core pain. See your pain as pure energy that's accumulated excessively over the years, which you are now going to begin releasing. I suggest that these people begin learning what it means to exercise emotion with a sense of finality. This is saying two very important things. First, it says that we as a culture have been programmed to exercise our bodies and our minds. Fitness, exercise, and looking good are extremely important to many in our culture. Exercising the mind through education is also a powerful theme in our culture. Yet when it comes to exercising the human heart, we are at a complete loss. It is seen as an obstacle in the way of our drive for material achievement. Furthermore, no one wants to be reminded of their own stored, repressed heartache by observing yours. So when it comes to exercising body and mind, we're all in. But when it comes to exercising our emotions, count us out.

The second message my statement offers is that when people do have a handle on releasing their emotions, they tend to forget that there can be an endgame. You and I have the power to sit down in a quiet room, feel the pure energy of an emotion, and release it with the sense that when we get up from the chair to leave the room we can be done with that emotion forever. It's a mere concept, but a very powerful one. Merely thinking that we are going to really let it all out with the intention of releasing every last drop of any given emotional energy has great power. It represents power that we are not accustomed to having. All transformational change begins with a change in our thinking.

Whole Health Suggestions for Emotional Overeaters

1. Begin thinking of your eating disorder as a heartache disorder that you have begun to associate with food consumption.
2. Choose to begin feeling your pain out, rather than feeding it down.
3. See your emotional pain purely as energy that has built up in excess, and nothing more. Your commitment is simply to release it.
4. Affirm that you have the power of closure over any given emotional release. You can, and will, complete the release of your emotional pain.
5. Never be afraid to seek professional assistance. It represents a source of support for your personal transformation. You will always remain the most vital source of true power in your own life!

CHAPTER 7

WHOLE HEALTH MIND BALANCING

PLACEBO/NOCEBO: THOUGHT DRUGS

During my earlier years of practice, I thought that optimal wellness was mostly about nutrition, but as time went on I began to appreciate just how multidimensional human health really is. I would soon discover the complexities and dynamics of the interconnections between spirit, mind, and body. Like many at that time, I knew that T'ai Chi, meditation, and yoga lowered stress hormone levels and relaxed the nervous system, but I became interested in the details. All at once, it had become very important for me to better understand how life-threatening stress was communicated from thoughts and feelings to cells and tissues. The prospect of a spirit dictating to the mind, the mind dictating to the brain, and the brain dictating to the body compelled a great sense of wonder in me.

I started to figure out that dis-ease often results when a rebellious spirit separates the mind from the body. I have witnessed a thousand patients violate their hypoallergenic diets by giving in to some pleasure food they were uncontrollably obsessed with. A rebellious spirit can easily coax the mind into the notion of instant gratification. Meanwhile, the victim body is forced to go along for a rough ride. The body may not have the same decision-making power—or voice—that the mind does, but it will eventually speak in its language of symptoms. And when the body speaks its pain, the spirit and mind are forced to listen. Pain is the voice that reminds us that the body, mind, and spirit are inseparable.

A man once walked into my office, sat down, and proceeded to explain to me that he had a rare condition whereby if he as much as thought about hot, spicy food, he would almost instantly break out into an acute full-body rash. He pointed out that his condition became chronic nine years earlier after having consumed an overdose of Trinidad Moruga Scorpion chili peppers, reputed to be the hottest of any pepper. From that time on, his thoughts alone were more than enough to trigger a terrible rash. Of course, I'm sure you know what comes next. I asked him if he felt comfortable with the idea of demonstrating this phenomenon. Sure enough, the man closed his eyes, visualized himself eating a hot spicy chili pepper, and within a matter of seconds, right before my eyes, his entire body broke out in a bright red rash.

I think of myself as a pretty accomplished problem solver, but you can be sure this gentleman's quandary put my abilities to the test. My natural instinct was to avoid going the way of the pill. My sense was that his body imbalance was rooted in his mind, and therefore he'd require a little neural pathway reformatting. I asked the man to close his eyes and take three slow, deep breaths. I wanted to guide him into an alpha brain wave state. Together, we could then create a visual image in his mind so that every time he thought of anything spicy he would immediately imagine a frigid, icy, snowy day. We further associated a great chill all throughout his body with the newly programmed image. We taped our brief session, which lasted for approximately fifteen minutes. He was instructed to listen to the tape twice daily for ninety days, and then return for a follow-up visit. He returned three months later and reported that his condition had been completely reversed! He learned that what his mind had been trained to expect is exactly what he got. We merely retrained his mind to expect a new result.

EXPECTANCY

I feel most fortunate to have come upon a remarkable story that appeared in the April 19, 2011, issue of *Psychology Today*, authored by Pamela Gerloff, entitled "The Possibility Paradigm: Transformational Change for Individuals and the World." Gerloff recounts the story of an overweight, forty-year-old teacher named Lester Levenson, who was diagnosed with a heart condition and told he had only a few months to live. His condition was so advanced that he was told by his doctors that even attempting to tie his shoes could be life-threatening. Paralyzed by the fear of dying, Levenson decided to deeply examine his every option. It clearly wasn't safe to move his body, but he could certainly move his mind. He concluded that deep unhappiness and negative thinking were among the causal roots that he could safely and instantly begin addressing. He began ridding himself of every negative thought pattern he'd ever had, and soon attained a state of what he called "imperturbability" (enlightenment). Within just a few short months, Levenson's heart condition was medically cleared, and he was declared completely healthy. Moreover, the state of mind he'd attained miraculously empowered him to heal other people and fix broken objects, by merely believing them to be "perfect."

Inspiring his students to inspirational levels of consciousness, Levenson would encourage them to remove all self-imposed limitations. They began to note that many of the lofty visions they'd discussed in class actually started happening to them. Levenson created a contagion of positive expectancy, for himself and for those around him. Thought expectancy generates a powerful flow of energy that is communicated from the spirit, to the mind, to the brain, to the nervous system, and to the immune system. Even the world of science has begun to discover that reality begins and ends with expectancy.

Noted Harvard psychobiologist Dr. Walter Cannon reported on a number of perfectly healthy tribal subjects who died soon after having been cursed by voodoo witch doctors. Cannon found that the reasons for death were ultimately the subject's belief in the spell and their certain expectancy that death would soon follow. To put it succinctly, when it comes to placebo (healing thoughts) and nocebo (harmful thoughts), what you've been trained to expect is exactly what you tend to get. It seems that our sense of reality is affected by our cultural beliefs and rituals, as well as by the perceptions and beliefs we share with our culture. Cannon reported that most voodoo deaths typically occur within one to three days and that the cause of this death was of psychobiological origin. The past forty years of placebo/nocebo research suggests that factors such as emotions, moods, language, ritual, attention, imagery, cognitive processing, and planning all greatly influence the placebo/nocebo effect. Studies have demonstrated that those inculcated in environments where negative thinking predominates are more inclined to nocebo tendencies, whereas those raised in more positive mental environments are more inclined to placebo effect. Yet another wave of studies suggests that one who is previously programmed into a negative cultural persuasion can be reformatted into a positive placebo mind-set. Thoughts alter cells. Expectancy alone has demonstrated its proven potential to produce marked changes in human brain chemistry.

In 2002, Emory University researcher Dr. Helen Mayberg administered PET (positron emission tomography) scans on mildly depressed subjects. Her study revealed that regardless of whether the subject received the antidepressant drug Prozac or a placebo, the same regions of the brain were activated. Patient expectancy can activate brain chemistry in a way that simulates actual drug treatment. The human brain is a powerful pharmacy that responds to the prescriptions written by our thoughts. Researchers Fabrizio Benedetti and Martina Amanzio of the University of Turin have performed studies on the neurochemistry of medical rituals. They have discovered that the rituals of Western medicine alter the neurochemistry of the brain in much the same way as tribal rituals. They've discovered that the expectancy of medical effectiveness is often more than enough to engage the healing effect. The smell of the hospital, the doctor's language, and the confident anticipation of results all make a significant difference in the placebo response. The research suggests that the same holds true for nocebo. Expectancy appears to be the medium for both placebo and nocebo chemistry, and the nature of expectancy begins with tribal ritual (or family system, in the Western sense) downloading. Cultural and environmental programming set the tone for our belief system to expect either good or bad outcomes. What we expect mentally, we receive physically.

My tendency has always been to use every healing tool available to me. Having rejected pharmaceutical power, I learned early on to rely on the intention of the spirit, the energy of the mind, the neurology of the brain, and the biochemistry of the body. From the very start I worked tirelessly to set a tone of positive expectancy. It became clear to me immediately that there were powerful, transcendent mental determinants at work that were more than capable of influencing overall health. True from the beginning as it is today, many of my patients routinely overcome conditions that the medical establishment insists they don't have the ability to recover from.

In 2010, I coproduced a minidocumentary (now accessible on YouTube) entitled *Choosing to Live*. It's based on six remarkable patient recovery stories—prostate cancer, breast cancer, multiple sclerosis, lupus, rheumatoid arthritis, and nonalcoholic cirrhosis of the liver. The minidocumentary came about because so many of my patients demanded a forum to tell their amazing stories. I have hundreds of patients still waiting to share their "impossible dreams." This joint effort is determined to show the world the uncharted possibilities of healing. As a culture, we have a difficult time grasping the power of positive placebo. But there is a well-documented history here that began more than thirty-five years ago.

In 1975, University of Rochester psychologist Robert Ader conducted an experiment designed to train rats to develop an aversion to saccharin-flavored water. First, Ader gave the rats saccharin water, and soon after drinking the water, the rats were injected with cyclophosphamide, a drug that causes extreme nausea. Much to Ader's surprise, many of the rats died. After tireless investigation, Ader eventually learned that not only does cyclophosphamide produce nausea, it's also a very powerful immunosuppressant. Thus, he tried giving the rats saccharin water without a follow-up cyclophosphamide injection. Nevertheless, the rats still died. He was amazed to discover that by programming the rats to behave as though the drug were in their systems, he had inadvertently taught them to suppress their own immunity whenever they drank saccharin-sweetened water.

One of my favorite placebo/nocebo stories involves a physician named Bruno Klopfer. In 1958, he was attending to a terminally ill cancer patient named Mr. Wright. The patient had overheard the doctor having a discussion about a new experimental "miracle" cancer drug. Wright begged Dr. Klopfer for the miracle medicine, but Dr. Klopfer refused, saying that it required more trials. Wright pleaded until Klopfer finally gave in. By all previous accounts,

Wright wasn't expected to live more than two or three days, as his cancer was quite advanced.

The drug, called Krebiozen, was administered on a Friday. Dr. Klopfer fully expected to come in that next Monday morning and be notified of Wright's passing. Instead, what he saw that Monday morning was Wright walking around in his room with a broad smile on his face. After further investigation, Klopfer wrote that in a mere three days, Wright's grapefruit-size tumors were "melting like snowballs on a hot stove!" A few days later, Wright was sent home, cancer free.

After two months, Wright remained cancer free—that is, until he read an article in his local newspaper reporting that researchers had discovered that the Krebiozen was being dropped from research due to trial failure. Within two weeks of reading the article, Wright was back in the hospital with his cancer returned.

This time Dr. Klopfer had a plan. He informed Wright of a new, improved form of Krebiozen being studied that was considerably more powerful and, initially, more effective in trials. Wright received injection treatments immediately, but unbeknownst to him, the only thing Dr. Klopfer was injecting him with was saline solution and sterile water. In two weeks, Wright's cancer had vanished, just as before. And for two months he remained cancer free until he'd heard a television report that Krebiozen had again failed trials and was being dropped. Wright died two weeks later. The spirit of the mind informs the brain, and the brain informs the body.

My father loved to tell a nocebo story related to his orientation week in the navy. Early one morning his squad was marched to the medical facility for their group inoculations. He said that the line was as long as the eye could see. As the line started to feather down, those men who had already received their shots were walking by the waiting line with pained looks on their faces, holding their ailing arms. As those men continued to pass by, they told the men waiting in line that the needle was frighteningly long, and as time went on, more men passed by the waiting line with increasingly exaggerated stories about the dreaded needles. Dad said that after thirty to forty minutes of having their anxieties inflamed, a number of the men waiting in line actually started passing out. When it came time for my dad to receive his shot, he was not surprised to find that the needle was actually quite small. I can still hear my dad's words: "Those men who passed out in line were merely victims of their own fearful imaginations."

In *The Biology of Belief: Unleashing the Power of Consciousness, Matter, and Miracles,* author Bruce Lipton writes about a British physician named Albert Mason. Back in 1952, Dr. Mason tried hypnosis to treat a fifteen-year-old boy who was afflicted by what was believed to be a severe case of warts.

Dr. Mason's initial session with the boy focused on one arm. Mason put the boy into a trance and told the boy that the skin on that arm would heal and turn healthy. Two weeks later, when the boy returned for his follow-up appointment, Dr. Mason was thrilled to see that the arm had drastically improved. But soon, Dr. Mason brought the boy to the referring surgeon, only to learn from the surgeon that what he was suffering from wasn't warts at all, but a potentially lethal congenital condition called ichthyosis. By attaining the miraculous results with hypnosis alone, Mason and the boy had done something that had never been done before. The hypnosis treatments continued until the boy's skin completely healed. Soon thereafter, Mason wrote about his treatment experience in the *British Medical Journal.*

His article created such a stir that patients from all over the world who were suffering from the disease descended upon him in search of his miraculous treatment. But Dr. Mason was never again able to reproduce the same results. When questioned about it some years later he said that, after learning of the mistake in diagnosis, he lost confidence in the plausibility of the treatment. As a classically trained physician, he was willing to accept the possibility that hypnosis might help cure a rash, but he didn't believe that it could treat such a radical condition—even though it *had*.

You may recall the "biology of belief" story briefly mentioned earlier in the book, about the art teacher who beat cancer by refusing to give in mentally. As I see it, she strengthened her body's immune system with the power of her mind.

Over three decades, I have learned from so many of my "patient teachers" that there is an unlimited power within us all, which is waiting to be channeled from spirit to mind to brain to body, and all activated by mere thought.

HIGHER MIND OVER MATTER

The mid seventies was a very transformational time for many of us. My brother's near-death experience set me on a new life path and inspired me on a search for deeper meaning. Enter spiritual study, meditation, and yoga.

Before too long, my study, meditation, and yoga had started to expand my higher consciousness. They were taking me to places in my mind that I'd likely been to many times before, only now I had a far greater awareness about where I was than ever before.

Each time I closed my eyes and went deeper within, I'd arrive at the inevitable question "Who am I?" You can only close your eyes so many times before your inner vision makes you wonder about the distinction between self that is *seen* and self that is *seer*.

I was awakening to a whole new perspective. After years of focusing on the outside world, I was beginning to discover an infinite world within. The concept of "self" was taking on an expanded meaning. There, within the universe of self, I was beginning to discover a silence flowing with information, a darkness radiant with light, and an emptiness filled with meaning.

Spiritual study, meditation, and yoga were becoming much more than mere exercises to lower my stress hormone levels. They were sparking a new interest in previously unexplored domains of higher consciousness.

I immediately began tapping into the infinite potentials of spirit within mind. I also had the good fortune at that time to study with some very special teachers who taught me how to master the greater power within. It was during this time, with their assistance, that I first came to understand the contribution such mastery could make to the prospect of doctoring.

It has always amazed me how profoundly we influence one another with the power of our intentions, thoughts, and words. Mere words alone can, in fact, inspire life or death. I point to a famous nocebo story that reportedly took place at a Catholic hospital in Washington, D.C., some years ago. As the story goes, a priest gave the wrong man, who happened to be healthy at the time, his last rites. A few moments later, the man died.

This "voodoo effect" often makes me wonder about the potential nocebo power of the physician's negative bedside manner. What about the power of a doctor's words, and the effects those words could have on their patients? Can a doctor's negative expectations be felt and absorbed by the patient in a way that affects their health? And can a doctor's disturbing words have the voodoo-like effect of a death sentence? How much dis-ease is caused by unconscious doctoring?

Spiritual study, meditation, and yoga had dramatically altered my sensitivity to consciousness doctoring. Never before had intentions, words, and actions meant so much. Suddenly I found myself paying very close, conscious attention to thoughts, dialogue, and choice of words. It had become very clear to me that the way I talk to patients might indeed make a significant difference in the outcome of their recoveries. I also began listening much more closely to patient dialogue. Were they thinking and speaking in terms of ease or dis-ease? Ease and dis-ease are born within the spirit of the mind, and they are reflected in the expression of every thought, word, and way.

I once received a very meaningful secondhand compliment from a patient. He told me that the associate of a very dear friend of mine, a Chinese healing master, was overheard talking to the master. He said, "Master, I am convinced that one of the reasons why so many of Mark Mincolla's very ill patients experience such great recoveries is that he is so positive, they can't bear the thought of disappointing him."

THOUGHT POWER

The brain is a biological organ. Each area of the human brain is highly specialized. The amygdala and hippocampus contain the circuitry that transmits anger, anxiety, and fear. The left prefrontal cortex is the area of the brain designed to facilitate logic and positive belief. The striatum is the processing center that mediates between these two divergent centers. As powerful as all this specialized machinery is, scientists have long wondered whether it's the actual machinery or the intricate programming that ultimately determines our positive or negative tendencies.

Researchers know that brain circuits can rewire themselves in order to adapt to new thought patterns, in essence rewiring new "happy" circuits in areas previously wired for "sadness." Our thoughts and, more specifically, our internal dialogue determine our wiring.

Recent neurological studies have shown that every thought produces a matching chemistry, and that each thought carries with it the capability to alter the brain and body. In a number of these studies, scientists have wired subjects to brain scanning devices to get a brain wave baseline. Those with very little "positive" left-brain prefrontal wave activity are instructed to repeat positive mantras such as "I am healthy, I am happy, and I love my life," ten minutes a day for twelve to sixteen weeks. At the conclusion, they are rewired. As you might expect, most of them rewired the "positive" left prefrontal area of their brains. Whether they're true or not and whether we believe them or not, our thoughts produce matching chemistries. Science has confirmed that if our dialogue is positive, then our brain will wire positively, and if our dialogue is negative, our brain will wire negatively. Our ability to wire our minds and brains for positive outcomes is without limitation.

I remember my dear friend Master Tom Tam once telling me that it was his common practice to balance the energy (Qigong) in the room he was about to present in, while en route to a seminar. Energy is everywhere, even a seminar room full of patrons. He'd project the mental intention to balance out negative attitudes, distractions, and bad energy that might be in the room where he was scheduled to appear. That way, the ch'i in the room would be favorably balanced out long before he arrived. Clearly this is one good reason why Tom's events always turn out to be so upbeat and successful. My seminars and media presentations have greatly benefited from his advice ever since.

Once while driving to the Fox 25 studios in Boston to appear on my weekly television segment, I decided to make my arduous morning commute a bit more productive by engaging in a simple but powerful neuroplasticity exercise. I repeated my own positive mantra for one solid hour. The mantra I opted for was one that was both very positive as well as a little shocking to the nervous system. I wanted to make sure my mantra really got my brain's attention. The mantra I chose was "I am the master of the Universe!" Remember, mantras needn't be accurate or truthful. They must, however, be positive and shocking in order to be neurologically attention-getting. It's all about generating powerful energy with word power, and I surely generated an hour of power!

As I entered the studio, the first thing I noticed was that the entire crew was significantly more energized than usual. There was a very playful spirit that one couldn't help but notice among the news anchor, the weather guy, and even the camera crew. Could the energy that I generated on the drive have really made a difference? One thing is for sure—I felt great! I also did the best segment I could ever remember.

My sister routinely views my weekly segment, so I typically call her immediately after it airs, as I can always trust her honest opinion and constructive criticism. Following this particular segment she remarked on how uncommonly spirited we all were. It seems my Qigong had indeed had a powerful effect!

Intentional thought patterns program the unconscious mind to invoke its power over certain levels of brain specialization, chemistry, and ultimately our perceptions. Willful energy can clearly alter material reality.

Master Mantak Chia teaches an ancient energy healing technique called Smiling into the Organs. It is exactly what it sounds like. The practitioner of this healing exercise closes their eyes and visualizes a smile in their mind's eye. Once clearly envisioned, the smile is then transmitted through the mind's intent to each vital organ, one at a time—to the liver, the heart, and all of the other vital organs, until the entire organ system has received "smile energy." This exercise goes back thousands of years and has truly remarkable powers capable of changing the landscape of one's day-to-day reality.

Several years ago, I was asked to deliver some public addresses in Palm Springs, California. I was listening to an NPR radio broadcast while driving to the auditorium and happened to catch a report on a study of the ancient Chinese smiling exercise. Sure enough, researchers from California had studied the effects of the exercise and discovered that the exercise had produced demonstrable health effects on subjects over a mere sixteen-week period.

Research such as this has helped us better understand the flow pattern of energy in the form of thought as it transits from spirit to mind, brain, and body. And when speaking about the human spirit, mind, and brain, we must not forget about the human heart.

THOUGHTS FROM THE HEART

The mind, brain, and heart are constantly in dialogue, paving the way for both miracle and disaster. The Centers for Disease Control estimates that 90 percent of all annual doctor visits are stress related. The St. Louis Behavioral Medical Institute says that 43 percent of all adults suffer adverse health effects from stress. By adverse effects, they are referring to heart attack, stroke, asthma, irritable bowel syndrome, Alzheimer's, Parkinson's, multiple sclerosis, rheumatoid arthritis, and the common cold, to name just a few. Thoughts and emotions are powerful energies that assert a great force on the human body.

With a vision of helping the world to better understand the mind/body connection to stress, Doc Childre founded the Heart-Math Institute in Boulder Creek, California, in 1991. HeartMath has since grown into an internationally recognized research and education organization dedicated to helping people reduce stress.

HeartMath researchers have discovered that the heart is an electromagnetic powerhouse, producing the strongest electromagnetic field in the body. They've found that the heart's field is 100 times more electrically powerful and 5,000 times more magnetically powerful than the respective fields of the brain. Over the years their studies have established that, when healthy and in balance, the human heart is electrically "coherent." Cardiac coherency is described as a state of rhythmic equilibrium generated by positive emotions. In other words, positive thoughts and emotions balance heart rate, blood pressure, and respiration rate. When stress generates negative emotions, the electromagnetic field of the heart loses coherency, and health is diminished.

HeartMath studies have determined that the heart is an intelligent, thinking organ. They have discovered that the heart has a "little brain," or cardiac intrinsic ganglia, that can think and communicate with the big brain. The heart not only knows what's going on—it tells the big brain what's going on. It sends messages to the brain about quality of life, happiness, contentment, and stress. The big brain then relays these messages to the body's global physiology. The heart is the central synchronizing mechanism in the human body.

Stress produces an energetic ripple effect from the inside out, from the mind's thoughts to the heart's little brain, to the big brain, and to the body. It begins as an event, or perceived event. I say "perceived event" because as we have seen, all you have to do is think about, or dream about, something stressful to engage the mind/body stress machinery. Once the mind registers and reacts to the prospect of getting fired from the job, crashing into the car in front of you, or running from an angry dog, stress becomes physiologically engaged via the mind, the heart's brain (intrinsic cardiac ganglia), the big brain, the nervous system, and finally the entire physiology, where health is then affected. This transmission of force from the mind's thoughts and emotions to the body's cells is engaged by highly charged bioelectricity, which generates an equally charged electromagnetic field. This is when you can actually feel your hair stand on end, as the energy in your body courses with adrenaline.

Virtually everything in the body, including the fight-or-flight stress response, depends on vital proteins in cell walls to regulate the flow of electrically charged atoms or ions—such as sodium, potassium, and calcium—between the interior of the cell and the surrounding fluids. This succinctly describes the bioelectricity of the human body that represents "the spark of life." It is in this way that stress chemistry is mediated in the human body. Stress and the coherent equilibrium of human health is mediated from mind to heart and from brain to body via bioelectricity and the electromagnetic fields it generates.

The human heart's electricity has been measured at 696 Hz, and the brain's at 315 Hz. The electricity of heart ECGs is sixty times greater than brain EEGs. The electromagnetic field of the heart is generated by every heartbeat, where it both produces and responds to a quantum field of information within and without, beyond the limits of time and space. There is a physiological heart, and there is an energetic human heart. The physiological heart is where stress and incoherency become a problem. The energetic heart is a transcendent field of consciousness intended by nature to be the solution for stress and incoherency. Within the energetic heart is a little brain with a higher mind that has the power to set the tone for our life's coherencies and incoherencies.

MENTAL EUTHANASIA:
THE ULTIMATE INCOHERENCY

It was a raw, rainy September morning in 1983. It was just another day at the office, or so I thought. Sitting before me, my first patient of the day was a woman who appeared to be in her early sixties. I'll call her Marion. I reached for my intake forms to begin recording her health and diet histories when Marion suddenly began to speak.

"Don't bother taking any notes. I don't intend to be here very long," she said. I knew instantly from the tone of her voice and the intention in her penetrating presence that the "here" she spoke of wasn't just my office. As I put down my pen and notes, I asked her to please continue.

"I've been diagnosed with an incurable form of cancer, and sent home to die," she said. "The only reason I've come here is because my children and grandchildren implored me to do so. You see, they believe that my life is about to end when, in fact, the truth is it never really quite got started."

At this point, it was clear to me that she was here to deliver a "sacred life lesson," and knowing full well that these do not come around every day, she had my complete and undivided attention. She continued, "As a young girl I was very distressed at how controlling and intimidating my parents were. They made all my decisions for me, and rarely allowed me the opportunity to express any of my opinions or true feelings. I remember feeling different than everybody else. I felt as though there was something wrong with me. I was deeply ashamed and figured I must have been undeserving of the kind of life all my friends seemed to have. This smothering control my parents had over my life predominated throughout every major event in my life, even to the point where they arranged my marriage. I do not, nor did I ever, love my husband, yet I remained loyal to him, to my parents, and to my indelibly subservient lot in life. Now, here I am, an old woman who never took charge of the life I'd been given, and quite frankly I'm just too tired to carry this old body around anymore." I just sat silently and listened.

"Don't get me wrong," she quickly added, "I do love my children and grandchildren very much. As I said earlier, the only reason I came here was to put on a good face for them, but the final fate of my cancer is not entirely unwelcome. So, you see, none of them will ever know the truth."

With that, Marion looked me right in the eyes in a piercing manner and asked, "Isn't it odd that I've come here today to share my most painful truth with you, a total stranger?" Knowing full well that she wasn't about to allow me the opportunity to enter into any healing pact with her, I simply told her I was honored to be entrusted with her story, and asked if there was anything at all that I might do for her. She told me there was one thing. . . .

"In your work, you will, undoubtedly, encounter many other people who never really took charge of their own lives," she said. "I would ask you to share my story with them, and to implore them to discover what it truly means to be self-empowered and fully alive." Marion died shortly thereafter, but her spirit will forever live through me as I continue to honor her sacred request.

Like Marion, many of the patients I see continue to remind me that healing is indeed the by-product of wholeness, and wholeness requires that we take full responsibility for our own lives, regardless of the demands. Moreover, the real lesson in Marion's tragic story is that by confronting our short-term pain, we liberate ourselves from the prospect of all long-term suffering.

THE WORD ACCORDING TO US

For years, I was an avid long-distance runner. I successfully completed a number of marathons, half-marathons, and ten-kilometer races. Now I am a dedicated four-season long-distance walker. I recall an occasion when I was walking near my home and, as is often the case here in New England, a stiff headwind impeded my intention to traverse up a steep hill. At first, I chose to personalize my struggle, as I muttered under my breath, "The universe must be conspiring against me." I mean, after all, there I was trying to do something healthy, like take a nice brisk walk, and the fates decided to throw this wall of wind at me. I'd unconsciously drifted into some all-too-familiar victim behavior. As the headwind intensified, my attitude also intensified. "What sort of sadistic beings are in charge of the weather anyway?" I mused.

Just as my tension peaked, something in me snapped, and my attitude radically shifted. All at once, I started to envision the headwind as a sort of giant air hose sent down from the heavens to blow away all my transgressions. Within a matter of seconds, the harder the wind blew, the *stronger* I felt. I could feel a surge of energy lifting me up and pushing me through the wind and up that hill. The very force that held me back just a few minutes earlier had suddenly been transformed into a power that propelled me forward. The mind *is* a reality-maker, and perception *is* a reflection of choice.

Rewiring the brain begins with changing the mind, and changing the mind begins with changing our thoughts. It is much less about what we believe and much more about our inner dialogue. The conscious mind is said to process more than 2,000 bits of information per second. Remember when I told you earlier that the *unconscious* mind can process more than *400 billion* bits of information per second?

Depending on what expert you listen to, research suggests that most of us average between 1,000 and 3,000 thoughts per minute. Not only do our thought directly affect our brain function, our inner dialogue alters our brain chemistry. A positive inner dialogue produces happy thoughts which produces a healthy neurochemistry, and a negative inner dialogue produces sad thoughts, which produces an unhealthy neurochemistry. When you consider all the thoughts and all the bits of information being processed in the mind, it's a bit overwhelming thinking about the chemistry changes. And it never ends. Even while dreaming, we produce correlating chemistries. Even the most cartoon-like nightmare will induce biological changes like sweating; heart rate changes, and dry mouth, while many a happy dreamer has often awakened laughing out loud.

The mind's thoughts and visions have a powerful influence over the body. Whatever we think and talk to ourselves about the most, we become. If we wish to change our lives by changing our thoughts, we must understand that belief is secondary. What you believe is important, but it's far less important than what you say. What you say to yourself has the greatest power to alter your destiny.

The Whole Health tuning exercise discussed in chapter 4 gives us all the information we'll ever need to know about the power of words. Like everything in the multiverse, words are energy. Word energy has the power to create ease or dis-ease. Our nervous systems determine exactly what neurological value a given word has, and word power depends on perception. For example, the word *cancer* generally has a negative neurological value for most people. Yet I can remember a gentleman I once muscle tested who'd been diagnosed with cancer. When I attempted to EMT-tune him, I called out "Cancer," just prior to muscle testing him, but instead of weakening the man, the word made him stronger. He explained that he was so determined to fight the disease, the mere mention of the word inspired his strength. A word that is generally a negative, weakening word for most, only served to elevate one man's determination and strength.

We can see from this example that the unconscious and conscious minds tend to correlate words with experiences. Thus, the positive or negative perception associated with a word often influences the neurological value of that word. Our words are responsible for our health, happiness, and prosperity. Reality is based on the word according to us.

WORD WIRED

Until 1993, it was a widely held belief that the brain we were born with is the brain we'd die with. Since the groundbreaking research of Peter Eriksson and Fred Gage at the Salk Institute, however, we now know that the human brain isn't hardwired. Rather, it is "neuroplastic" and designed for constant change; the human brain can be neurologically rewired and the mind can be reformatted. Moreover, it doesn't demand miracle drugs or surgery—it merely requires word power. One of the most respected pioneers of neuroplasticity research, Dr. Richard Davidson of the University of Wisconsin, reminds us that our words produce a matching chemistry—not our histories, our belief systems, or our philosophies, but our words.

Words generate differing neurological power, as they represent varying powerful images. The word *lonely* will momentarily weaken the electromagnetic field in our heart (cardiac intrinsic ganglia), while the word *happy* will strengthen it. As the heart's brain conjures up a positive or negative image associated with whatever word is presented, the nervous system begins producing a corresponding chemistry. Depending on the image the heart's brain associates with those words we hear most often, the brain will either produce a "fight-or-flight" or a "relaxation" response. Thus, your neurological chemistry is directly correlated with the images generated by those words you speak and hear the most. If your inner dialogue and the dialogue of those you spend most of your time with exhibits a tendency to be negative, your neurochemistry will likely generate a negative influence over your entire physiology. We are word wired.

WORD REWIRING

The most inaccurate phrase in the human language may well be *I can't help it.* Beliefs such as "My mother was a worrier, therefore I will always be a worrier" die hard. We've heard so much about genes and genetic determinism over the past thirty years that we're inclined to believe that hardwiring indeed equals fixed fate. After all, human genome research has long since established that you can only change a gene $\frac{1}{10}$ of 1 percent every 250 generations! I routinely hear from patients that their physicians tell them their respective health conditions are the result of genes, and that short of medication there is nothing they can do. Much of the medical community continues to toe this line. And while it may be a great "point of sale" for the pharmaceutical industry, it is no longer as enthusiastically embraced in the genetic research community. Many of those who once accepted that the human brain was hardwired and the human body/mind couldn't be changed all that much have altered their viewpoints.

We may only be able to change our genes one-tenth of 1 percent every 250 generations, but we now know that we can change the behavior of our genes, and to initiate the process takes only seven-tenths of a second! The dogma of molecular biology that embraces absolute determinism has been shattered by new research. We also know that influences such as nutrition, emotions, thoughts, and beliefs regulate the expression of genes. Every cell membrane has receptors that pick up an array of signals that influence the ways in which we translate and adapt to our internal and external environments. Where we once believed that our brains and bodies were hardwired, we now know that words alone can rewire us. We are in fact not hardwired at all—we are neuroplastic.

The most recent research has made it clear that words alone have the power to set both patterns of biocoherency or incoherency into motion. Each word produces a unique energy that transmits waves of vibration that can be received by the cardiac intrinsic ganglia. Next, the heart's little brain determines whether or not the word represents an energetic vibration that produces electromagnetic entrainment or disentrainment. Once determined, the little brain then conveys its verdict to the big brain, where it then communicates it to the rest of the entire body via the nervous system. Researchers have found that in order for the heart to return to a state of coherency during times of destabilizing stress, words alone are often more than enough. Not just any words, but positive words. When it comes to the cardiac intrinsic ganglia, every word we speak or hear has a different value. Energetically speaking, every word produces a different vibration. Some words produce an energetic coherency, and others an incoherency. So it's not just about what a word says—it's also about the energetic vibration of the word.

Ultimately, when we allude to electromagnetic fields, we are of course talking about vibration. Sound and light waves represent the most fundamental forms of kinetic vibration. Therefore, one sure-fire vehicle for affecting the vibration of the heart is sound. As most of us have heard, music soothes the savage breast. But even more than words and songs, sounds and tones alone will elicit a powerful effect on the heart's electromagnetic field. We must choose our words wisely.

ERASE AND REPLACE

Over the years, I have done a good bit of corporate wellness and nutritional consulting with Fortune 500 companies, and have administered positive thinking programs that I've documented with noteworthy results. I once instituted an Erase and Replace program. There were two tasks that I asked of subjects in this program. For the first task, I asked hundreds of corporate associates to mindfully tune in to and consciously register all negative inner and outer dialogue. They were instructed to immediately erase all negative dialogue in their mind and replace it with a positive word or phrase. If a friend complained about the snow and cold, I instructed them to tell a white lie. They were told to say to themselves that it was sunny and warm. Remember, it's all about word power!

For the second task, I asked associates to spend ten minutes a day for twelve weeks reciting the following phrase: "I am happy, I am healthy, and I love my life." Many of the subjects asked if it mattered that they really didn't feel the emotions of the words, and didn't believe what they were asked to repeat. My answer was, "It doesn't matter what you think or believe. Just keep repeating the words. Words alone have rewiring power. Your brain will ultimately accept the energy associated with the words you speak. What's more, the positive word power will be passed on to your nervous system." Sure enough, that's exactly what happened.

At the very beginning of each program, I asked each of the subjects from the Erase and Replace group to fill out a detailed questionnaire regarding their state of mind and emotion. I wanted to know quite a bit about them. Were they ever diagnosed with depression or anxiety? Did they frequently experience mood swings or feel out of control? Did they feel powerless or struggle with the notion of accepting responsibility for their own lives? I also wanted to know if their mental and emotional tendencies affected their quality of life at home and/or at work, and if so, in what way?

After repeating the phrase, "I am happy, I am healthy, and I love my life," for ten minutes a day, every day for twelve weeks, the results were as follows:

* 64 percent said they felt less depressed;
* 63 percent said they felt less anxious;
* 71 percent said they felt more in control of their thoughts;
* 71 percent said they felt more in control of their emotions;
* 86 percent said they were more aware of negative thinking in those around them;
* 100 percent said they felt more empowered in their lives;
* 100 percent said they were more focused on their goals;
* 100 percent said they felt more hopeful in attaining their goals;
* 100 percent said they felt more inclined to accept full responsibility for their lives;
* 100 percent said they intended to continue practicing what they'd learned in the program.

Once again, it's what your brain hears most that makes the difference. Your words generate an energy that influences your thoughts and formats your nervous system. Want to improve your overall well-being? Pay conscious attention to your words. Focus on creating a constant stream of positive inner dialogue. Remember, your brain was designed to reflect how it is programmed!

We tend to resist change, even though we're designed for it. It's a matter of positively adapting our thoughts so as to support the messages from our mind to our brain. Decide exactly what you want, and in what ways you'd like to change. Map out your desired changes and then distill your vision down to a word mantra, like the example you read about from our group program. Then continually rehearse it over and over every single day. Remember, the more positive and shocking your mantra, the more likely it is to get the attention of your nervous system. You must compel your nervous system with the power of your words.

Your mind will signal the program change to your brain, and your brain will encode it into your neurochemistry. Soon you will come to experience a transformational reality shift. Your mind talks to your brain, and your brain is your relay center for physical change. It has 100 billion neurons that make 100 trillion communication connections. These connections determine and reflect personality, knowledge, character, emotions, memories, beliefs, and dreams.

THINKING YOUR WAY TO A LIFE "IN PURPOSE"

Any force that's denied flow will result in disharmony. Cholesterol blocks the flow of blood to the heart. Repression blocks the natural release of human emotion. Ultimately, both will result in dis-ease. In much the same way, if denied our true authenticity and higher purpose, we will be forced to contend with the same unfortunate outcome.

The amount of energy it takes to *not* live your life "in purpose" can drain the very life right out of you. I have seen tens of thousands of patients crippled with the fear of such a risk. All risk must be qualified. There are dangerous risks and there are calculated risks. I am not referring to dangerous risks here. I am speaking about calculated risks associated with the advancement of our higher destiny. Such natural risk-taking can be profoundly empowering. Any vision of great success must carry an equally great risk of failure. These risks represent the very challenges and lessons that we came here for. They are the source of our most sacred "tension." The tension that we so often curse is, in effect, the blessing that can only become transformed by our willingness to take the risk.

I try to remind myself to celebrate my tensions when they arise. I believe that the sooner I celebrate them, the sooner their transforming effect will take hold. Tension is merely fuel that propels spiritual growth. Only my distorted fear of risk-taking can hold me back from living my life "in purpose."

Living a life in purpose can actually alter our chemistry. It allows life force to flow more freely and abundantly within us. As long as we remain open, and trusting of our deeper instincts, we'll live in a more inspired, homeostatic state. Living a life in purpose unleashes powerful healing forces within. Entering into such a state of personal solidarity, our endorphins drive up our production of neuropeptides, which then dramatically increase our immunological strength. Conversely, I know of *no* cure for *not* living a life in purpose.

So often, I hear people say that no matter how hard they try, they simply can't seem to get in touch with their life purpose. Many are frustrated, and even burned out over the prospect of such a challenge. Still others even feel that not everyone was designed to get in touch with such weighty stuff.

The ancient Chinese sages believed that each and every one of us was given a specific life purpose. They believed it to be secretly hidden, like a treasure, directly behind the heart. They believed that the only way to discover it was to direct your awareness into, and ultimately right through, your heart, until you arrive at this treasure on the other side. To those who say they can never know their true life's purpose, I simply say, it's time to begin your journey through to the other side of your heart.

LIVING BACKWARD: A TRANSFORMED MIND, A HIGHER PURPOSE

The two and a half years in my life between March 1, 1992, and December 31, 1994, was nothing short of cataclysmic. It all began with my father's sudden, unexpected passing. Nine months later, on the very same morning my youngest daughter was born, I was jolted by the news that my fifty-three-year-old brother, Anthony, had left this world without warning.

As the months passed, my family and I were so overcome with grief that we were desperate for any hint of serendipity that might bring us together for an occasion other than a funeral. As providence would have it, my twenty-six-year-old nephew, Michael, was to be wed to his lovely fiancée, Rachel, in October 1994. This was just the window of fresh air that we needed. It was a magnificent celebration that uplifted us all and made us feel as though we were at last coming out of what had seemed like an endless tunnel of darkness. Things were beginning to settle back into place for my family. Then, a mere two months later, on New Year's Eve, my sister, Rhonda, called to tell me that Michael had just died from an anaphylactic reaction to medication. Only two months after his wonderful wedding celebration, Michael was also gone. As a family, we were beyond gone. When I say "we," I would include everyone left standing in my family except for Rhonda. By all accounts, my sister was holding it together. At all the wakes and funerals, it was Rhonda who remained steadfast and strong. Even after the loss of Michael, her firstborn son, she remained stoic.

A few months after Michael's funeral, Rhonda took the train to New York to visit our cousin Mary. As the train pulled into Penn

Station, Rhonda suffered a sudden heart attack. For months Rhonda underwent an endless battery of blood and stress tests. She was under the guidance and care of a very dear friend who, as luck would have it, just happened to be one of the world's most respected heart specialists. After all the tests were completed, the doctor requested to meet with Rhonda regarding her results. He told her that there was absolutely no logical biological reason that could explain her heart attack. Astonishingly, her test results were normal. He explained that this sort of clinical anomaly represented one-in-a-million odds.

"Rhonda," he exhorted her, "this is very difficult for me to say. I have only seen this in very rare circumstances, but I believe your heart attack may have indeed been the eventuation of your emotionally broken heart. In order to heal your physical heart, you must, at last, let out all your grief, for the greater good of your health."

In the days and months that followed, it was obvious that Rhonda was going through some dramatic changes. It had become clear to us that she was in the process of reordering her life. She had been forced at the hands of fate to "get real!" There was no room left to store her grief. In her reordering, she was forced to get in touch with all her deepest feelings, both good and bad, both expressed and repressed. As is always the case, pain and suffering paid a visit in order to deliver a life lesson. In this case, the delivery was made and the package was claimed.

Those of us closest to her knew full well that she was determined to get in touch with, and fulfill, the needs of her authentic self. She soon contacted me and requested that I design a diet and lifestyle plan for her. She also asked me to help her work out her spiritual and emotional conflicts.

I have never seen a patient so determined to attain true wholeness. Nor have I ever seen a greater commitment to self-discipline.

Her diet, her workout regime, and her self-discovery were firing on all cylinders, but you could feel that there was more to come. There were intangible, yet palpable, forces unfolding from deep within her.

Rhonda had been married for thirty-six years, during which she'd never known the burdening responsibility of being so awake. Now she was all too aware of her innermost feelings, and she was at last ready to take full responsibility honoring them. She arrived at the difficult conclusion that things had become far too stagnant in her marriage. Not bad, mind you, but stagnant. There was no animosity. There were no irreconcilable differences, just too much rust on the relationship. She demanded that she and her husband see a marriage counselor in hopes of reestablishing some dialogue, but dialogue wasn't the prescription for getting this kind of rust off. "I guess after thirty-six years of anything," she said, "humans tend to automate."

Following a period of counseling, Rhonda came to the conclusion that she needed to move on with her life. Some relatives and friends struggled mightily in their vain attempts to understand Rhonda's profound changes. Nevertheless, she remained unconditionally dedicated to her sacred process. I will forever respect my sister for her uncompromising courage.

Our sacred process is rarely understood, or approved of, by the world. Nonetheless, the spiritually strong always soldier on through their sacred process, one bold step at a time. Sacred process reveals two kinds of people: those who are *externally reactive*, and those who are *internally proactive*.

Externally reactive people are "other" directed. All too often, they are the victims of narcissistic deprivation. As patients, they're inclined to feel that they simply don't deserve to recover. Their sacred process invites them to wrestle their rightful power back into their own hands. But, for many, their fear of self-empowerment so impels them to yield to rigid demands of "other" and to keep peace that they end up depriving themselves of their own vital needs. Ultimately their drive for safety drains the life out of them.

Internally proactive people are "self" directed. Survivors of terminal illness are often transformed into internally proactive people. They are committed to living life fully alive, regardless of approval, opinion, or conflict. As patients, they tend to overcome their illnesses because they've learned well the art of living life "backward," in some cases by nearly losing it. They've found themselves on the edge of a precipice where they no longer have the luxury of indulging in self-denial. They have the distinct advantage of knowing what their ending looks like.

I often advise my patients to first look at their final step in life before trying to figure out their next step. I tell them, "Envision the final scene in your last chapter, then slowly work your way back, filling in all the blanks in the novel of your life, right back up to the present step that lies before you." After all, you are the author and the main character in the classic called *Your Life*. Always be fully mindful in the presence of each precious, unfolding chapter.

I've always considered every patient to be my teacher. Profound life lessons can be learned from those survivors who have walked to the cliff's edge and called themselves back. They are the true masters of the art of living life backward. They have much to tell us about looking into the nature of the whole selves we are all yearning to be.

In order for your life to be fully lived with authenticity, you must open the eyes of your soul. To do so, you must be willing to see the absolute truth. The soul's vision sees only the unedited truth. Its vision begins with the end of your life and works back to where you are. The soul's vision is the only thing that separates those of us who are destined for greatness from those of us who resist our greater destiny.

I have had the good fortune to have worked with a great many patients whom traditional medicine practitioners had given up on. They were sent home to make their peace with themselves, their families, and their lives. Yet, paradoxically, it was because they walked right up to the edge of no return that they were somehow able to generate an uncommon force of will capable of rescuing them against all odds.

I shall never forget one woman I worked with who was sent home to die with stage four breast cancer. She had three young children who inspired her to remain steadfast and determined to beat the dreaded disease. She did, and as she walked out of my office victorious on that glorious day, she turned to me, broke down in tears, and said, "I thank cancer for teaching me how to live." The disease of cancer has *taken* the lives of many, but the experience of cancer has also given life to some.

Living life backward provides you with a very different perspective. It reveals a vision of who you really are and what you really need. It reminds you that life is precious and fading fast. It beckons you to stop pretending that you have forever to postpone all that is most meaningful. Thanks to my terminally ill patients, I have come to believe that deep within all of us there resides a soul that generates life energy to the spirit that resonates through to our hearts. It is not a prerequisite that we walk the tightrope of near-death in order to be given the opportunity to be made whole. We need only learn the art of living life backward. When you get to the end, you'll find that . . .

There is no denial.

There is no pretense.

There is no illusion.

There is only naked truth, and a new beginning . . .

TRANSPECTANCY

Transpectancy is a word I created by combining *transformation* and *expectancy*. *Transformation* refers to a radical change of form. *Expectancy,* according to recent neuroscience, represents thought power that can actually change life-and-death outcomes. It implies the kind of thinking that fuels both placebo ("I shall heal") and nocebo ("I shall harm") potential. Thus, "transpectancy" is meant to describe *positive expectation with the power of drastic change*. Limiting belief is the primary obstacle that stands in the way of the power and potential of transpectancy.

Belief is merely thought that is empowered by mental and emotional states. Therefore, if I empower a negative belief with a negative mind state or emotion, I turn off the positive life-changing potential of transpectancy.

The Three Disablers of Transpectancy

There are three mind states that empower limiting beliefs and disable the potential of transpectancy:

1. *Fear*—"I feel too unsafe to expect positive outcomes."
2. *Shame*—"I feel too undeserving to expect positive outcomes."
3. *Doubt*—"I feel too disappointed to expect positive outcomes."

In the most primitive sense, the unconscious mind was designed to protect us by remembering and reminding us of all the negative experiences we have ever had, whether real or imagined. Whether dominantly programmed to trigger fear, shame, or doubt, the subconscious mind never forgets. It continues to believe in every trauma, nightmare, and negative thought. If a child never burned his hand on a stove, but his mother did when she was young, that child will likely be programmed to fear stovetops through the mother's negative subconscious programming.

Your most emotionally charged and repetitious thought patterns always shape your reality and, in the case of fear conditioning, it's a reality that binds and limits growth and prosperity. Those thoughts that fire through your nerve networks most often ultimately wire corresponding nerve networks together, reinforcing the same repeated thought patterns.

The key with transpectancy is to initiate new positive thought patterns until you become more willing to expect positive outcomes. The best way to begin establishing new, positive thought patterns is through neuro-associative conditioning.

Neuro-associative conditioning (NAC) is a well-studied technique that has proven that you can actually reshape your reality by reprogramming your nervous system through positive thinking.

It's quite simple. Your nervous system is neurologically wired to respond most dominantly to two variables: pleasure and pain. You can actually alter the reality dictating nerve network chemistry in your brain by replacing old pain-based thought associations with new pleasure-based programs. In the case of the child and the hot stove, as he matures, he might think of how much he enjoys certain favorite meals. As he begins rewiring his belief system regarding stovetops, instead of thinking about the negative experience his mother once had, he can begin thinking about the potential of that stovetop to produce the pleasurable meals he enjoys so much.

When you rehearse linking positive experiences with events once believed to be negative, you rewire your brain's nerve networks in a manner that initially allows for, and ultimately reinforces, a greater tendency for positive expectancy.

Three Transpectancy Exercises

1. *Erase and Replace Exercise*—As previously discussed, the Erase and Replace exercise begins with making a commitment to living much more mindfully. Observe more consciously all that happens within and around you. Focus on your observations at a level of positive and negative. Note all the negative energy that comes from the minds and mouths of you and everyone around you. Edit out, or erase, all the negatives, and replace all

forms of negatives with positives. Every word you speak and every thought you think creates a matching chemistry! Your reality is your choice!

2. *Positivity Exercise*—Take four minutes twice daily to repeat a simple positive, shocking mantra such as "I am a genius." Turn off your cell phone and don't listen to any music during your commute to and from work each day. This will likely ensure you the time required. In my ongoing neuroplasticity work with patients over the past ten years, I've discovered that by taking just four minutes twice daily for sixteen weeks, you can significantly develop the left prefrontal cortex (the positive, confident mind). Your brain and neurobiology do *not* know the difference between what you speak and imagine and what you actually experience. It's all processed the same way in the anterior cingulate cortex of your brain. This is why nightmares can increase your heart rate. Your brain takes your mind's thoughts and spoken words literally. Thus, your reality (including your physical health) is programmed by your brain, and is based on what your mind dictates. All the research indicates that our brain programs everything based on what is most frequently repeated in our thoughts.

3 *Tibetan Manifest Exercise*—This particular version of a 3,000-year-old exercise comes from the John Perkins book *Shape Shifting: Shamanic Techniques for Global and Personal Transformation.* The exercise was handed down to John from a European traveler, who learned it from Tibetan sages. The sages told the traveler that "it will most assuredly make dreams manifest!"

Begin by closing your eyes. Keep your eyes closed until you complete the exercise. Next, envision your intention. Now envision the black void of space all around you. Then picture a bright, shimmering silver star at a distance out in front of you. Project your intention through your third eye (which resides in the middle of the forehead) out to the silver, shimmering star, where it will then be absorbed by that silver star. Once the star has absorbed your intention, draw the silver star containing your intention into your mind through your third eye. Now, picture that the star filled with your intention explodes three times in succession within your mind. These are transformational growth explosions. They are expanding the power of your vision. Following these three growth explosions, direct the silver star containing your intention down into your heart. Once again, imagine three powerful growth explosions in your heart. Finally, draw the silver star filled with your intention up and out of your third eye, back out into the black void. Perform this exercise at least twice each day, three times per week.

TRANSFORMATIONAL VIBRATIONS

In January 2012, a team of astronomers from the University of Arizona reported that they had detected the actual original sound waves from the Big Bang, believed to represent the birth of the universe some 14 billion years earlier. Big Bang theorists postulate that the universe expanded from the size of a proton particle (smaller than a grain of sand) to macrogalactic proportion. Every bang creates sound, and some theorize that the Big Bang produced "the primordial" sound. The University of Arizona team of astronomers says that stars and galaxies actually formed along the ripples of those first sound waves, where the matter was denser. The important point is that sound waves were among the first natural vibrations that resulted from the birth of the universe. Sound produces a cosmic vibration.

Since the dawn of civilization, sounds, tones, and overtone harmonics have been considered sacred agents of healing. There is evidence of healing with sound, in overtone healing chanting traditions in Bulgaria, Central Africa, China, Japan, Native America, Romania, South America, Spain, and Tibet. Harmonic tones were often combined with mantras, or "words of power," for the purposes of attaining spiritual transcendence and healing. Buddhists, Celts, Christian Mystics, Hindus, Jews, Muslims, Sai Babas, Sikhs, Sufis, and Taoists all had mantras and chants to elevate their spirit, balance their nervous system, and heal their ailing bodies.

Over the centuries, each culture established its own relationship with healing sounds. In all cases, overtones and words of power (mantras) are revered as sacred sounds with the vibrational potential to significantly relax our nervous system and elevate our energy. The Hindus embraced the mantra *aum*, believing it to represent the primordial sound. The Buddhists often employed the mantra *tat tuam asi so ham*, which translates as "thou art that I am." The Taoists have employed five healing sounds for more than 5,000 years. Each is believed to have the power to heal a corresponding major organ of the human body when recited with frequency. The sound *ssss* (pronounced *shee*) is believed to heal the lungs. *Wooo* (pronounced *chwaaay*) is for the kidneys. *Whooo* (pronounced *whooo*) is for the spleen. *Shhh* (pronounced *hsuuu*) is for the liver, and *hawww* (pronounced *herrr*) balances the heart.

PERSONALIZED SOUND MANTRAS

We all produce our own unique energetic vibration. Our vibration is like our DNA. You can't change it, but you can decipher it and, once you do, you may then employ its extremely powerful energy-balancing and healing effects.

While reciting traditional sounds, words of power and mantras are effective ways to tune one's vibration. Whole Health teaches that we each have a specific sound of power that, once discovered and recited with regularity, will elevate our vibration response to a far greater level than ever before.

Whole Health has developed a system called the personalized mantra protocol. Over the years, Whole Health has tested and calibrated sounds and has discovered that vowels have all the power. Consonants have nowhere near the vibrational energy that vowels do. Therefore, this system implements only vowel sounds. Whole Health has also established that, in order to increase the power of mantras by personalizing their vibration, the subject's individualized musical key must be determined.

We are all energetically and, thus, vibrationally unique. Therefore, the concept of dialing in the vowel sounds and exact musical keys from person to person with specificity is what makes the Whole Health personalized mantra protocol so very powerful. There is a simple EMT muscle testing exercise that will enable you to decipher your own personalized mantra.

Before beginning this EMT exercise, you must access a Personalized Mantra Assessment (Appendix D). You are also advised to perform this exercise with a partner. Next, assume EMT pass/fail posture. Then commence tuning and establishing reliability (for a review of these exercises, see chapter 4).

The practitioner and subject must set their intention to reverse the polarity. This simply means that when they arrive at the correct positive response, instead of strengthening, the subject's arm weakens and drops down. It is important to reverse polarity whenever there are many variables to be tested, as it will prevent arm fatigue.

Next, the practitioner must call out all the vowels one at a time—A, E, I, O, and U. Only one of the vowels will cause the subject's arm to fall. This establishes the subject's personalized mantra vowel.

Next the practitioner calls out the seven musical keys (one short of an octave) one at a time—A, B, C, D, E, F, G—muscle testing the subject's strength response with each key called out. When the subject's arm falls at the practitioner's calling out of a specific key (and there will be only one), you have established the musical key (tone) of the subject's specific personalized mantra.

Now you can establish the amount of time that the subject's

mantra must be recited. The practitioner calls out time intervals from one to ten minutes. As always, when in reverse polarity, once the subject's arm drops, you will have established the recommended time allowance for them to recite their personalized mantra. The practitioner should also test the subject for the number of times the subject should recite their personalized mantras per day. Personalized mantras are generally never to be recited for less than one minute once a day, and for no more than ten minutes twice a day.

In the calibration process, Whole Health has discovered that, on average, the personalized mantra protocol increases one's personal vibration millions of times more than the average traditional mantra. This is in no way intended to diminish any sacred mantra. Traditional mantras have a great history, and are often aligned with sacred traditions. The Whole Health personalized mantra protocol is intended to assist in elevating the energy of one's vibration, and will surely do so.

PERSONALIZED VISUAL MANTRAS

This very powerful exercise is designed to energetically balance the spirit by establishing a subject's receptive sensory dominance, as well as their visual nature mantra. We all have our own unique sensory affinities. The concept of receptive sensory dominance suggests that we each resonate energetically with one or more of the specific five senses. Whole Health says that once we establish the dominant innate sensory nature of a person, we can help them cue into those specific sensory images to balance the spirit. For example, if we wanted to help someone with stress-induced hypertension, and their dominant senses were sight and smell, we could have them visualize a beautiful beach and imagine smelling the fresh salt air.

Neurolinguistic Programming (NLP) is a truly remarkable school of thought that has developed numerous effective protocols for the positive reformatting of the negative unconscious mind. NLP's implementation of submodalities, or sensory images, has been shown to produce incredibly powerful, positive shifts in unconscious thought and learning. The more graphically and energetically you engage the mind, the easier it is to gain access to fertile areas where new seeds of thought can be planted so as to replace negative old self-limiting thought patterns.

The Five Sensory Submodalities

1. Visual (Seeing)
2. Auditory (Hearing)
3. Kinesthetic (Touch)
4. Olfactory (Smell)
5. Gustatory (Taste)

This spirit-balancing exercise begins with the practitioner EMT muscle testing the subject for their receptive sensory dominance. Interface, assume pass/fail posture, test for reliability, and tune. Then, the practitioner simply calls out each of the five senses one at a time as they pass/fail test the subject. Next, the practitioner must pulse test the subject from one to ten. The subject's strongest response (with the highest pulse number) represents their receptor sensory dominance.

Next, the practitioner must test the subject for their visual nature mantra. Along with the Five Sensory Submodalities, Whole Health lists Seven Visual Mantras.

Seven Visual Mantras

1. Ocean/Beach
2. Lake
3. River/Stream
4. Waterfall

5. Desert
6. Forest
7. Mountain

Next, the practitioner must pass/fail and pulse test (from one to ten) the subject for their most energetically responsive visual nature mantra. The visual mantra that pulse tests the strongest will offer them the most powerful energy access to spirit balancing.

Then the subject must take two minutes to engage in a combined sensory nature visualization. For example, I muscle test them for their sensory kinesthetic response to the visual imagery of a forest. So my spirit balancing is easily attained when needed by simply imagining myself touching the dewy ferns, pine needles, maple leaves, and rocks in one of my favorite wooded areas. Following two minutes of this sensory nature visualization, the subject should be tested for the degree of improvement of their spirit balancing. Do so in percentages. Example: "As a result of this spirit-balancing exercise, the subject's spirit energy balance has improved by [then pulse test for 10 to 100 percent]."

Our many spirits reside within our mind. As with our body, we must cultivate balance within our mind in order to attain and maintain a state of true wholeness. Like the body, the mind requires daily feeding and exercising to be healthy and whole. Every mind is but a reflection of what thoughts it is fed and the manner in which its energies are directed. State of mind is the result of choice and development.

BALANCING THE MIND AT THE ROOT SPIRIT

As we have previously discussed, the prefrontal lobes are the parts of the human brain primarily involved with long-term planning, personal evolution, and the attainment of internal goals. With the aid of positron emission tomography (PET) scans and magnetic resonance imaging (MRI), neuroscientists have in recent years made further discoveries about how the left prefrontal cortex is centrally involved in the implementation of positive goal-oriented behavior, while the right prefrontal cortex processes signals that convey a sense of threat—often resulting in inhibition, fear, and anxiety. There are also ongoing experiments in transcranial magnetic stimulation of the left prefrontal cortex that continue to consistently demonstrate mood improvements.

There is a distinct difference between these two vital brain centers. In order for our long-term planning to reach full fruition, there must be a balance between the two lobes. Research is revealing that dominance in the right prefrontal lobe is typically associated with limiting blockages of emotional thought that keep one from moving forward with their life goals, breeding further fear and anxiety. In short, an imbalance between the lobes, especially one that results in right prefrontal dominance, represents a greater likelihood of your getting stuck in your own mind. There is no debate over which comes first. Depressing, self-limiting thoughts create brain imbalances, and brain imbalances create depressing, self-limiting thoughts. It works both ways. Therefore, the cycle of being broken spirited and stuck in life can be rewired with the aid of positive thinking and positive inner dialogue. Over the years I've gotten remarkable results with a number of personally developed positive dialogue protocols, but I've also had great success with some specific Chinese energy healing techniques. One of these is called Balancing the Root Spirit.

In Chinese medicine, the acupuncture points for the right and left prefrontal lobes of the brain are the Gallbladder (GB 13) points (bilateral). They are referred to as the "root spirit points," and are located right in front of each prefrontal lobe at the edge of the hairline on each side of the forehead (see Figure 7.1)

Whole Health's Balancing the Root Spirit exercise is very simple. It begins with EMT muscle testing, so it is recommended that you work with a partner. As always, you must interface, assume EMT pass/fail posture, establish reliability, and energetically tune. Assuming your prep work has been completed, you are ready to begin.

First, practitioners must pass/fail test the subject's right and left GB 13 points by lightly touching each area or by simply calling out, "Left gallbladder 13," followed by "Right gallbladder 13," one at a time, and testing the subject's arm strength. Test their muscle strength simultaneously as you call out the respective points. Next, practitioners must pulse test the points in plus/minus numbers. Now record your results. These results represent the subject's energetic prefrontal lobe dominance. Remember, if they are weak while being tested on the right side, it means there is excess emotion blocking the spirit's desire to flow. If they are weak while their left side is being tested, it means there is a deficiency of emotion resulting in a lack of passion needed to propel and inspire spirit flow. Next, it's time for balancing the spirit root with Wenchiech'u.

While interfacing, practitioners should simply spin counterclockwise spirals with their index finger or their thoughts and in-

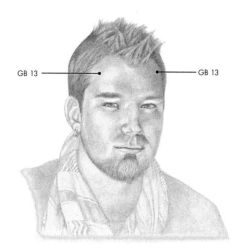

GB 13 — GB 13

FIGURE 7.1   GB 13

tentions over the deficient areas for two minutes. Next they should spin clockwise spirals over any lobe area that may have tested with excess energy for two minutes. You have now balanced the root spirit. Encourage the subject to repeat this exercise on themselves twice daily, every day, for two minutes. After a few months, subjects will experience dramatic positive changes in their thinking, confidence, and personal growth. Once balanced at the spirit root, the brain and mind are also in balance.

CHAPTER 8

WHOLE HEALTH SPIRIT BALANCING

THE SPIRIT QUEST

We of the modern West are at a distinct disadvantage in matters of the spirit. Our material culture struggles with concepts that elude the five material senses. Nonetheless, our pain has always been at the ready to teach us more about our deeper nature.

I have counseled many in search of solutions to help shut off their "pain switch." I am quick to remind them that physical symptoms are, in fact, the language of the body, and that it's important for them to trace back their inner pain dialogue from their body back to their mind—and even further back, to their emotions and spirit. Pain represents the surfacing of our deepest communication with ourselves. I advise them to tap into what their outer pain is trying to tell them about the innermost nature of their imbalances. Physical pain isn't the end of the discussion among our body, mind, and spirit—it's only the beginning. Our physical pain initiates a dialogue that ultimately leads to the root source of our spirit's dis-ease.

I ask them to take one giant step—a quantum leap—beyond where the present pain manifests. I advise them to resist the temptation of numbing their pain. I remind them that it's essential to follow the voice of our pain to where it leads us. Our "pain voice" has designs on leading us on a journey deep within ourselves to the roots of our present suffering. The very pain that forces us back to the roots of our dis-ease is the catalyst for our spirit quest. It is part of "the way of things" for pain's destructive nature to inspire us back to our creational source. The natural dis-ease process is initiated at the very instant of our separation from spirit. The further we drift away from our spirit essence, the louder our pain voice gets. You might say that dis-ease and pain are a spiritual fail-safe. Just as spiritual separation lies at the root cause of dis-ease, our physical pain is the alarm that awakens us and directs us back to our core spirit identity.

A dying patient once requested my presence at her home on the evening she passed. I shall never forget how she went in and out of physiological consciousness, and as she did she rambled in a most peculiar manner. Then after quite some time out of consciousness, she suddenly opened her eyes, looked up at me, and said, "You know, Mark, I feel as though I'm at last discovering who I truly am." She took her last breath soon after, but her words will forever remain with me.

SPIRIT "I"DENTITY

Many years ago, I was inadvertently inspired to decipher the deeper meaning of the biblical phrase "I am that I am." Of course, I'd read and heard this reference countless times, but never considered that there might be hidden meaning in it. On this particular occasion I was guided to intensify my concentration on the phrase, and I arrived at a very different understanding than ever before. I was inspired to place the emphasis on the word *that* instead of the words *I am*. It was as if the divine voice was awakening me to the fact that it was *that* I am—the one that no one is paying attention to. I could suddenly see that the words *I am* had been distracting me from the power of the word *that*.

This epiphany inspired me to contemplate the concept of universal duality more deeply. In this case we're all represented by both a human "I am" and a divine "I am." I began to realize that this simple biblical riddle may have been intended to liberate us from the nightmare of our guilt, shame, and self-contempt, and invite us to a better understanding of our own true spirit, or "I"dentity. It brought me right to the razor's edge of my own duality. I have a divine "I am" within me, living side by side with my mortal "I am." I tend to get lost in the illusion that I am purely mortal, and that the concept of divine refers to something other than me. There is no "other"—"other" is an illusion. There is only oneness. Together, my divine self and my mortal self make up my wholeness.

Personal "I" misperception is the distortion that evokes the destruction that results in dis-ease. Discovering our immortal "I" and integrating it with our mortal "I" represents the quantum leap to transformational wholeness.

I recently spoke with a patient during a phone appointment who seemed to unconsciously slip into a trance as she repeated an endless loop of self-limiting phrases, "I am sick," "I am overwhelmed," "I am afraid," and so forth. After a few minutes of this, I decided to interject. I asked her to take the time to consciously identify her core "I." I wanted to challenge her to reexamine that place from within her that generated her true "being-ness," versus her thoughts, images, words, and beliefs. I suggested that as she searched out the source of her "I," she consider choosing between a creative power and a destructive force—as we all have an ego and spirit self. I further explained that she might consider thinking of her destructive

"I" not as a conscious manifestation of evil, but as an unconscious misidentification.

I reminded her that we can choose to live our lives consciously, or unconsciously, from our higher or our lower self, and in an integrated or a dis-integrated way. Spiritual exceptionalism is always an option.

Quantum mechanics theorizes that between any two divergent domains there's a wave function collapse—a place in between two contrasting realities where everything stops. Similarly, between the zones of our mortal and our immortal consciousness, there lies the peace and stillness of unconditional self-acceptance. We can either perceive our dual nature as torment or we can take a quantum leap into the void of peace between our divergent selves.

CREATION/DESTRUCTION

On any given day our spirits can be high or low, depending on what we encounter and how we translate it. Our spirit's perception of the vicissitudes of life traces back to our core belief system. If we've been programmed to think of everything as either being good or bad, then we're likely prone to react to life's highs and lows conditionally. Succeed, and our spirits are high—fail, and they're low. Unfortunately this dualistic perception leads to a dead end, as the multiverse in which we live is dualistic and therefore infinitely tension-bearing.

Creation and destruction represent the eternal dance between power and force in the multiverse. Power is energy that both creates and results from order. Force is energy that creates and results from chaos. Every conscious and unconscious thought is an act either of creation or of destruction.

Our thoughts, dreams, wishes, visions, interpretations, actions, and non-actions are all either creative or destructive. We are forever producing ease, or dis-ease with all our creating and destroying.

The powers of creation and the forces of destruction are reflected in all our life choices as well—the foods we eat, the music we listen to, the books we read, the movies and television programs we view, and the company we keep. We are constantly cultivating either creative power or destructive force.

Being the sensitive receiver that it is, our spirit remains attuned and open to the constant formatting of our reality. But our spirits are often vexed by the highs and lows of mortal life. It is therefore important that we develop a higher understanding of the mutual compatibility of opposition. It's a matter of conscious choice whether we dwell on the extremes, or on the balance point between the two. We might think of ourselves as spiritual surfers catching a ride between perilous waves. To balance artfully on our board, we learn to benefit from the propulsion of the waves' power. Losing concentration, however, will likely result in disaster.

The great Chinese philosopher Chuang Tzu reminds us that together, creation and destruction make up one whole. He points to the visual exemplification of this in the T'ai Chi Circle, which graphically reveals the balance produced from the opposition between all universal extremes. The light is perpetually flowing into the darkness just as the darkness is perpetually flowing into the light. It's all about perspective. The Western mind is generally drawn to the illusion of separateness between the light of creation and the darkness of destruction. By separating the two, and perceiving one as good and the other as bad, we create a reality of dis-integration.

The ancient Chinese myth of universal creation begins with total chaos. As the whirling tumult settled, it formed the cosmic egg of creation. A primeval giant named P'an-Ku was believed destined to become the architect of the universe, but could only be born after the cosmic egg of creation cracked in two. The key lesson in this legend is that creation could not result without destruction.

A young woman once asked me the secret of healing her broken heart from a recent relationship breakup. I suggested that she envision her experience as being on hold. "It isn't complete yet," I told her. "Your experience will remain incomplete until you're ready to welcome in what it cleared a space for." I reminded her that the destruction of this breakup was merely clearing the way for the creation of her next experience. She was of course resistant at first, insisting on clinging to the force of her own destructive pain. I told her that she was clinging to destructive pain only to infuse emotional meaning into her life. Finally, I reminded her that she had the power to create positive meaning, if she would only come to understand the balance between her creative and destructive potential. Sure enough, she contacted me no more than a month later and thanked me, saying that she'd found her way into a new and more balanced relationship. "Ever onward," I responded.

Dis-ease isn't about destruction, it's the result of imbalance, and healing isn't about creation, it's about cultivating life force from the tension between the two. Creation and destruction are like two hands forever pouring life in and out of us. Embracing this reality brings a lasting peace to our spirit.

EASE/DIS-EASE

Energy is either positive, negative, or balanced. When our spirits are balanced, there is ease. When our spirits are imbalanced, there is dis-ease. Though energetic, our spirit interacts with our material glands and organs. The lower kidney region is the energy zone where our need for safety, security, grounding, and confidence resides. We might think of this as our "ease center." The adrenal glands (or upper kidney region) are the energy zones where our emotions of fear, fright, and panic reside. This represents our "dis-ease center." Ease produces the energy of flow and disease produces resistance. When the spirits flow, there is a sense of peace that transmits a parasympathetic relaxation response to the nervous system, which generates homeostasis and whole health. When the spirit is ill at ease and resistant, it transmits sympathetic fight-or-flight energy to the nervous system, producing dis-ease.

We all have both a mortal and an immortal will. Our spirit represents our immortal will. It has an affinity for non-action and unconditional peace. The mortal will of our ego produces conditional reaction and tension. Here, we can clearly see the exposed roots of ease and disease.

I was once scheduled to give a presentation at a karate school that was owned and operated by my good friend and three-time gold medalist, Chris Rappold. I felt it might help my presentation if I knew a little more about the origins of karate. It's a philosophy that believes in a higher force that can only take possession of the hand of the martial artist when they clear out a space and invite it to act through them. Belief in a higher universal order is essential to the ease of spirit. The multiverse is ordered. Creation and destruction are one. Without understanding "the way of things," our spirits can't hope to attain a balanced state of "ease."

THE T'AI CHI BALANCE

Classical Chinese medicine tells us there is but one true source, and two manifestations of all things. That's to say that everything comes from one unifying point of origin, but has a dual nature. Expansion and contraction, creation and destruction, and birth and death all serve as reminders of the ever-present duality that defines the multiverse.

We, too, are both rational and intuitive, temporary and infinite, ego and spirit—moreover, we are both human and divine, capable of anger and forbearance, jealousy and forgiveness, hatred and love. Our very duality is most often the cause of our greatest frustration. We often find ourselves torn between our greater and lesser angels. But the greater our confusion, the greater the expansion of our consciousness must become, and the greater our consciousness, the more empowered we become. Great wisdom is born of the greatest confusion.

The ancient Chinese Taoists capture this concept in a symbol called the *T'ai Chi Tu*. This visual icon, often referred to as the yin/yang circle, reveals a symmetrically arranged interposing of two semicircles, one black and one white (see Figure 8.1). It signifies the natural order and renewal of a multiverse that is continually regenerated by the tension of opposing forces.

Creativity and destruction, life and death, health and disease appear to us to be absolute opposites, but the T'ai Chi Tu symbol reminds us otherwise. The great circle of wisdom teaches that in an integrally unified universe, separation is but an illusion. All opposition produces regenerative energy. Furthermore, these cycles are not linear, nor are they static, but rather they are circular and fluid. These multiversal cycles of energy are forever shifting from one polarity back to the other. December 21 may be the first day of winter and the shortest day of the year, but December 22 represents the first cyclical shift toward spring, as the first day of increasing daylight.

I have seen these dualistic energies play out in my work with people as well. You may remember I once counseled a woman who

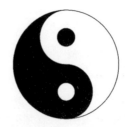

FIGURE 8.1   *The Tai Chi Circle*

was diagnosed with late-stage breast cancer. When we first began she explained that she'd been very repressed all her life. She described her father as a very imperative, intimidating person who discouraged her from opening up to her own power. As she described it, she was programmed very early in life to believe that she didn't matter. Subsequently, she found herself in a marriage and family where the same dysfunctional themes predominated.

Following a rigorous battle with the disease and a series of spiritual epiphanies, she was declared cancer free. Over the many months we worked together, it became very clear to me that her power was evolving through the inspirational challenge of her ordeal. At last, with great passion, she embraced just how much she really mattered.

As our final visit together concluded, she rose up from the chair and began to cry tears of joy and thanksgiving. She said that she would forever be indebted to cancer for teaching her how to truly live. She was emboldened by her victory to at last live her life knowing that she truly mattered, inspired by the very opposing force that once threatened to take her life away.

The great Taoist philosopher Lao Tzu taught that we come to escape the duality of birth and rebirth through the consciousness that understands that separation is but an illusion.

And so it is with our spiritual self, and our mortal self. We may appear to be made up of two very distinctly different selves, but in truth these two represent one whole and complete self. Only through higher consciousness can we decide whether or not they are unified and aligned.

The same fire that can burn us can also warm, feed, and protect us. The same water that drowns also hydrates and sustains. The same self that's flawed leads to the perfected self. Most would struggle mightily at the prospect of placing a divine self and human self within the same circle. We have been programmed to believe in the polar opposition of these forces. We've been taught to understand God as a perfect and complete spirit, tucked away in some heavenly domain, far away from us and our shameful spirit nature.

For us, God has become an "external" concept that we file under the "other" category, while our perception of "self" remains isolated and eternally flawed. But there is no "other," nor is there separation; there is only oneness. If the T'ai Chi Tu teaches us anything, it is that everything in the multiverse is comprised of both "this" and "that." For most, imagining such a thing would be considered an act of spiritual heresy. Furthermore, it might require a level of self-love we don't feel deserving of.

IMMORTALITY CONSCIOUSNESS

Aligned with the teachings of classical Chinese medicine, the Whole Health Healing System is based on attaining and maintaining a natural balance between body, mind, and spirit. It is also about understanding that the natural processes of both ease and dis-ease are rooted in spirit. Moreover, ease or wellness may only be cultivated by the attainment of what the ancient Chinese sages referred to as "immortality." But their understanding of immortality was very different from ours.

The ancient Chinese didn't have to be reminded that they were not humans having a spiritual experience—they knew well that they were spirit first. Our modern material programming distracts us from realizing that, though human, we are of spirit nature. The mere fact that we are spirit implies immortality. Therefore we already have immortality, but it can only be actualized through spiritual cultivation that realigns our awareness with our spirit. To emanate from the innermost core of spirit is to cultivate ease and immortality. To emanate from our mortal ego, on the other hand, is to remain suspended in the state of dis-ease.

Self-cultivation through diet, exercise, spiritual development, and energy balancing was considered a prerequisite to living out one's full natural life cycle of 120 years. The main reason they strove to live so long was to attain spiritual immortality.

We are each forever immortal but can only attain immortality consciousness through Whole Health self-cultivation. The quest for immortality consciousness begins with balancing our body's spirits, or "waking up the organ spirits." Waking up the organ spirits is also a phrase that refers to energizing the separate spirits that exist within each organ. As you will see below, Whole Health has devised an acupressure technique for waking up the spirit of each organ. Each of these organ spirits represents a five-element influence.

THE FIVE SPIRIT BLOCKAGES

When our spirits are ill at ease, we become totally imbalanced and our entire being enters into the state of dis-ease. This is something that no one can deny. The ancient Chinese ascribed to the belief that each vital organ is vivified by a specific spirit that profoundly influences and is influenced by that spirit. They teach us that human emotion is a reflection of the vital connection between deep feelings and spirit.

Our culture maintains a very different stance. We are programmed to repress and deny emotions, as they represent a force counter to our material drive. Addiction and obsessive compulsion result from our inability to contend with the massing force of our emotional repression. There is even a dissociated awkwardness around our therapeutic approach to dealing with our emotions. We are inclined to medicate our emotional state. And even while engaged in counseling, we are told to let our emotions *out*. The fact is, we *are* our emotions. The only thing we can let out is the volcanic backlog of repressed energy from the unnatural resistance of who we really are. The ancient Chinese innately understood all this.

They knew well that the key to emotional wellness is to maintain balance. As with all things, this was done through the Five Elements Principle.

In keeping with the five elements, there are five positive and five negative emotions that exert the most profound influence over our spirits. In fact, as we shall see later in this chapter, there are five specific spirits within each of our major organs, and five corresponding sets of emotions that, when imbalanced, become the causal roots of our blockages. Blockages of any kind, especially of the spirit nature, will result in energy imbalances that obstruct our path to wholeness.

Painful life experiences, distorted perceptions, lack of emotional adaptability, and painful memories are among the key factors that initiate and reinforce our dis-ease-producing emotional spirit blockages. Each of the five sets of emotions generates very powerful ch'i that can affect a whole self for a lifetime. To live in a state of wholeness, we must first cultivate an energy balance within our organ spirit emotions.

The Five Organ Spirit Emotions

1. *Anger/Kindness* influence the *liver's* spirit balance
2. *Hatred/Joy* influence the *heart's* spirit balance
3. *Anxiety/Compassion* influence the *spleen's* spirit balance
4. *Grief/Courage* influence the *lungs'* spirit balance
5. *Fear/Calm* influence the *kidneys'* sprit balance

The key to Whole Health spirit balancing is to maintain a conscious equilibrium between the positive and negative emotions. We are not to numb ourselves to our true feelings, nor are we to become addicted to their powerful energy. We all suffer from emotional energy imbalances that are the result of excess and deficient expression—the objective is to clear these blockages so that our core ch'i can flow outward to our mental and physical bodies. After clearing the blockages, we must continue to consciously maintain a consistent balance of our emotions with the aid of the Whole Health techniques taught in this book. Before further elucidating on Whole Health's clearing and balancing techniques, it is important that we gain a clearer understanding of how our organ spirit emotions become imbalanced.

THE LIVER SPIRIT'S ANGER

The liver's spirit represents the immortal soul. It is believed that only when we master the balance between our anger and our kindness will we enter the threshold of our immortality. Life is hard and no human being can ever receive enough love. The frustration that gives birth to human anger requires no more than this, for a tainted will is easily violated. The planet has always known of the outward manifestation of anger and war, as humans have forever rebelled, sometimes violently, against anyone or anything that opposed or violated the intentions of their mortal will. And if ever we were to indulge our anger, our mortal will would stand in direct opposition to our own immortal will. But our immortal will is determined to guide us down the path of balance and wholeness in spite of the rebellious nature of our mortal will. Nonetheless, spiritual evolution is a process with great growing pains and, until we do grow up, misguided anger exacts a great toll. The destructive energy from malevolent anger is both acted out as well as acted in.

We are all part of the most material sociocultural experiment ever attempted. During our developmental years, we're conditioned to understand that winning alone is solely correlative with material entitlement. It doesn't take very long to get the message that losing is simply not tolerated. This highly competitive socialization may work well for some. For others it only seems to impose shame for what are natural inadequacies, and guilt for what are believed to be sins and failures. There may be good spartan or meritorious intent here, but over the years I've witnessed the profoundly disabling effects of such spiritless inculcation.

I've seen far too many people who, because they are saturated with discouragement, have simply given up on life. These discouraged and angry people often internalize their anger by engaging in unconscious self-destruction. I have met far too many who are capable of healing, yet refuse to do so. They've been unconsciously indoctrinated to believe that they're undeserving. Not everyone can be a winner, and chronic loss often leads to feelings of failure, guilt, and shame—and after a life of losing, the prospect of losing life seems a fitting ending. Initially they may have been angry and bitter at the world for depriving them, but eventually that anger and bitterness become internalized.

During my consultation interview I often ask patients, "On a scale from one to ten, with ten the highest, how deserving of a life of abundant health, love, and happiness do you feel you are?" It is truly astounding to hear their responses. Most take quite a while to answer, and then when they finally do, the number that they offer is often very low. No more than two people out of ten answer with a ten.

This little exercise often sparks introspection, and further in-depth conversation. Many are all too willing to discuss their binds to guilt, shame, and anger. Failure and inadequacy are natural facts of life, but far too many of us have become enraged inwardly from the resultant self-contempt. Failure, guilt, and shame fan the flames of the liver spirit's anger, blocking the light of love and self-love.

I have observed many terminally ill patients who were given absolutely no chance to survive miraculously will themselves to live—just as I have observed patients who had no business dying leave this world. All of this is due to the delicate balance between self-contempt (internal anger) and self-love (internal kindness).

THE LIVER SPIRIT'S KINDNESS

Lao Tzu once wrote, "By the accident of fortune a man may rule the world for a time, but by love and kindness he may rule the world forever." The ancient Chinese understood everything as energy. As was just pointed out, there is an energy associated with excess internalized anger that breeds illness. I have met many who suffer from inflammatory conditions such as esophageal reflux, migraine headaches, and cirrhosis that are rooted in internalized anger. You can actually feel a tense energy within yourself at the mere mention of the word *anger*. The word *kindness* generates energy as well. It produces a gentle healing energy when spoken aloud. Kindness and forgiveness present us with a healing way to be gentle with the self.

Many years ago, I befriended an internationally acclaimed psychic from New York who was noted for his work with the FBI. He was a brilliant man who put his psychic gifts to work solving crime cases, but he also had a very high spiritual IQ. I was in my early twenties and was going through some emotional growing pains at the time. I remember asking him what the secret was to finding true inner peace of mind and personal solidarity. Without hesitation he urged me to learn how to become gentle with myself. He emphasized that the most elusive of all spiritual gifts were kindness and gentleness toward self. I recall feeling a bit perplexed as to how to go about zeroing in on his spiritual prescription. Like so many, my narcissism was extremely underdeveloped. Through the years I continued to work at it, and now many years later I credit it with being the most important advice I was ever given.

We must keep in mind that the multiverse is dual. Separation is an illusion. The Ta'i Chi Circle is intended to serve as an ever-present reminder that everything, including you and me, has a mortal and an immortal nature. I often remind my patients who pray to stop praying outward and upward and to start praying inward and deeply downward. God is a resplendent energy that resides within, as well as without. We may be half human, but we are also half divine. Self-forgiveness is less difficult to conceptualize when you come to understand this. By design, we must both fail and succeed in all that we attempt. One of the greatest secrets of life is that life is not about attaining fleeting success—it's about gaining eternal wisdom. This is wisdom that results from our understanding of the sacred nature of failure, pain, and suffering. The zone of tension between success and failure is the divine catalyst that powers the multiversal dance of life. Self-contempt resists this life power— self-forgiveness invites its flow.

The ancient Chinese referred to the spirit of the liver as the Immortal Soul. Kindness brings an end to the contempt that prevents the immortal soul from delivering its precious life force to our being. The pain and destruction brought on by self-contempt disguise tension to appear as something negative. Tension must be thought of as a sacred catalyst that initiates destruction and consummates with creation. Tension from self-contempt is designed to bring us full circle from destruction to regeneration and self-creation. Kindness, forgiveness, and gentle self-reflection open the energy gate of the immortal soul, allowing for the flow of life-giving ch'i to awaken and resuscitate our being.

THE HEART SPIRIT'S HATRED

History has proven that one man's hatred has enough negative power to destroy civilizations. Nonetheless, Chinese Taoist wisdom reminds us that all emotions are natural, even hatred, and that dis-ease only results when there is an unnatural imbalance in emotion. It's not the emotion, it's the suppression of the emotion that leads to the excesses that causes dis-ease. The ancients felt that it was natural to hate evil people, addictive substances, or tragic events. In such cases, our hatred serves as a protective agent that keeps us out of harm's way. They advise us to honor all our emotions, and to consciously remember that they are merely energies that require constant balancing.

Our culture tends to sanitize emotion with drug, drink, and distorted belief. Many with whom I've met suffer from their illnesses in part because they have disconnected from their deeper emotions. We must remember that energy can neither be created nor destroyed, only transmuted. Therefore, when hatred comes up for us, it should be recognized as an energy that must be expressed externally, or else it will be internalized, increasing our likelihood of unconscious self-destruction. I advise my patients to demystify these deeper emotions, and to think of them merely as pure energy. When we become shamed, intimidated, or guilt-ridden over our natural emotions, we open the door to a flood of dis-ease-producing energy. This negative energy then masses and shifts its movement from spiritual and emotional to physical channels.

This is actually a perfect place to once again point out the paradox of duality. As we have repeatedly said, everything is a reflection of the T'ai Chi Circle and, as with all things in the multiverse, we are dualistic. We are both mortal and immortal beings. We are composed of dark and light energies, and as with yin and yang, our opposite manifestations are constantly flowing into each other. The tension of our duality was intended to result in our integrated oneness, for separation is but an illusion that results in dis-ease. The higher self clearly understands the mutual compatibility of opposition. Our divine consciousness knows that hatred naturally emanates from the spirit of the human self, even as joy flows forth from the spirit of the divine self. The tension that arises from our hatred does so only to get the attention of our higher consciousness. By paying closer attention to the tension, we increase our probability for solution finding. In this case, the solution is only arrived at by integrating our duality so as to naturally express our hatred, feel the resulting hurt, and heal the divide within. Destructive hatred can then be understood as the catalyst for the creational integration of self.

THE HEART SPIRIT'S JOY

The ancient Chinese referred to the heart's spirit as the Emperor. It's important to keep in mind that they believed their ruling Emperor to be a direct descendant of God. Thus, the spirit of our heart was thought to represent our "God self" and its divine joy. By cultivating true unconditional joy, we heal our heart's spirit, and our heart's spirit then fills us with abundant ch'i. Material joy is a conditional and temporary state reactive to the rising and falling vicissitudes of life. In this sense, one is conditioned to be joyful only when gratified. Love, money, and fun are among the many material prerequisites that allow for material joy. Spiritual joy is a state attained only by grace, or through spiritual cultivation. Neuroscientists are now saying that happiness is a learned skill and that, by retraining our thoughts, we can map out new nerve pathways that reshape the joy pathways in our brain. They also tell us that repetition is important. By continually rehearsing positive thoughts and perceptions, we give direction to our reality architects—the mind and brain—to construct a domain of unconditional joy. True heartfelt joy doesn't come naturally to most of those who've been raised in this highly conditional culture, but it can be realized through dedication to spiritual cultivation.

The title of my first book is *The Wu Way*. I adapted the spelling from the ancient Taoist philosophy of *Wu Wei*, or "doing without doing." This represents the highest wisdom, which suggests that there is abundant joy awaiting the seeker who allows it to get their attention. Wu Wei reminds us that within the silent depths of our immortal heart, there is a wellspring of joy that needs only to be left undisturbed. For only when we close our eyes, empty our hands, and silence our noise will we at last see, touch, and hear all of the true joy that has forever awaited us.

THE SPLEEN SPIRIT'S ANXIETY

When we live our life out of balance, negative reaction naturally follows—all pain demands a response. The manner in which we respond to pain parallels our level of consciousness. Ultimately, all human response to pain is either of a destructive or a creative nature. Our destructive reaction to pain generally manifests as an obsessive drive to distract from the hurt. Just make the pain stop, and make it stop now! Thus, our self-destructive nature is drawn to fast-acting substances that numb the nervous system from its sensory awareness of pain. This ego-driven approach to pain resolution is immediate and short term, setting the stage for addiction.

Pain fuels an insatiable demand for intense distraction that can only be attained by abusing overpowering substances. There is no end to this destructive cycle of pain management. Pain creates affliction that drives addiction. The only natural solution is to consciously get in touch with, and release, the stored destructive energy around our accumulated emotional pain. If the volcanic energy of our pain isn't externally released, it is destined to implode.

We've become an addictive society largely because we are so driven to generate pain. We've even managed to find ways to create pain at the treatment end. We get people off heroin only to addict them to methadone. Attend an Alcoholics Anonymous meeting, and you'll quickly get the idea that it's off the booze and on to the cigarettes, coffee, and sugar. Our dysfunctional health care system is having a hard time figuring out that our most painful wounds are rooted where it's unable to find them, deep within our spirits.

Our culture is fast becoming an assembly line expressly designed to manufacture bipolar imbalances. We tend toward the extremes of repression, acting out, depression, and mania. Our wanton suffering self has been subliminally programmed to want pleasure, and want it now. Our ego is of course resistant to all the spiritual lessons of pain—it seeks instead to disable the process where our lessons can become our blessings.

As we evolve in higher consciousness, we become better equipped to process our pain at a spirit level. The five organ spirits produce extremely powerful vibrations, generating ch'i that is more than capable of healing the imbalances created by deep emotional pain, suffering, and self-abuse. Only by filtering pain through the prism of spirit can the most painful lessons lead to the grace of wisdom.

I worked with a man who first came to me quite some time ago with acute asthma. As a small boy, his philandering, addictive father became the source of stress and lifelong grief, which brought on his inflammatory asthma. His instincts told him that the reason his condition never responded well to medication was that it was emotionally rooted. The deep roots of his suffering had spread from his past to his present and even into his future.

He explained that the stress between him and his father laid the foundation for a dysfunctional relationship with his daughter. He had a distorted perception that she'd taken his love for granted—and for this he harbored great resentment. The more we discussed it, the more he began to realize that his vexation about his daughter ran deeper than he'd suspected. In fact, we came to see that he was actually angry about having to be a father at all. He felt so abandoned during his youth that his inner child didn't want to have to compete with his daughter for attention. Subsequently his daughter's been in therapy for many years. It might seem like a depressing story, but they're both spiritually evolving from pain to gain together. The pain that destroys is the same pain that can create. Only spirit can make it so.

THE SPLEEN SPIRIT'S COMPASSION

Passion is a word that evokes a powerful visceral effect. If any word generates energy, it's *passion*. The word *compassion* is equally powerful. I've always said that compassion's energy is passion minus the fire. Fire is extreme yang, and indeed powerful, yet the weakest form of yin (water) is the most efficient way to extinguish it. The power of passion commands our immediate attention—the power of compassion tends to elude us. Compassion may be passive in the material world, but in the world of energy its power is truly great.

The Five Elements Principle teaches that only compassion has the power to distract the brain's anxiety signal. You could be experiencing great anxiety, but by simply shifting your anxious mind's thoughts to thoughts of compassion, you can greatly relieve your tension.

The ancient Chinese believed that the spirit of the spleen was the energy center for the Intellect. As the primary residence of our wisdom, the spleen is where we contend with the delicate balance between grounded reality and free-floating, negative imagination. Think about it: much if not most of what we worry about never happens, and some never really could. When balanced, the spirit of the spleen is the intellectual balancing point where we ground our thoughts. Compassion intellectually snaps us out of our negative imaginary delusions, bringing us back down to earth. Imagine yourself walking down the street filled with unrealistic anxieties. Your thoughts are spiraling out of control when suddenly you come upon a lost, crying child. The compassion from within your spleen's spirit compels you to "get real," fast! This child needs your help immediately! No questions asked, you're in service and all your anxious delusions are long gone and far away.

The human brain produces a number of different brain wave states, most of which are scientifically observable. One state in particular, called beta brain wave bursts, was once believed to be untraceable. That is, of course, until a group of Buddhist monks were recently hooked up to brain scans and observed. I described earlier how the monks engaged in what they called a compassion meditation, where they exercised powerful mental intention to send healing energy through the ethers to wherever it was most needed. Lo and behold, following the compassion meditation exercise, the scientists were able to observe beta brain wave bursts. It was determined that the traceability of the elusive bursts was due to the power of their loving intention.

THE LUNG SPIRIT'S GRIEF

Grief is energy that, if out of balance, tends to generate great hopelessness. Chronic, acute grief might be thought of as clouds of spiritual darkness that don't allow the light in. We've all been there. It's human nature to experience temporary grief from loss, or deep disappointment, but with some, grief is like being sentenced to life in prison.

I often explain to my patients that grief, like all emotions, is a natural tool provided to us by nature to help us with energy decompression. As the pain of loss hits, we build up intense pressure that the release of tears helps relieve. Studies have shown that human tears contain the stress hormones prolactin, adrenocorticotropic, and leu-enkephalin, which are all released by crying. At some point toward the end of our crying release, tears reveal higher concentrations of "feel-good" endorphins. The key point here is to turn the corner from the "feel-bad" part of grieving to the "feel-better" part. It's important that we try to grieve with a conscious intention to finalize—to go through the stages of grief only once and not repeatedly. It's called "natural healing."

As a culture, we are very awkward about emotion in general. We exercise our bodies and minds, but we are at a loss as to how to exercise when it comes to emotion. In the case of grief, it's very simple. Our hardships produce an emotional buildup that needs to be released. It's about quieting the mind and listening to the language of the heart. Only the heart can lead the way—but it is essential that we remain consciously in tune as it takes us on our emotional journey. We grieve, but we don't always do it with awareness and with an intention of finality in mind. Some continue to grieve over the same thing on and on and on. That's why so many people repress and deny their grief. They believe they will be uncontrollably overcome by the tidal wave within. They don't understand that they have the power to consciously predetermine when they'll be done, and thus to finalize their grief.

Every other aspect of our lives has a beginning and an ending. When we exercise our bodies, we do so for an allotted time, and we're not done until every task has been counted out and checked off. We exercise our minds the same way. We sequence our way from kindergarten through grade school, high school, and college on a calculated and timed basis. So it should be with our emotional exercise.

I advise my patients to set up their grief exercise environment in advance. Choose a place and time where you will not be disturbed. Put the Do Not Disturb sign on the door, and turn off the phones. Create an environment for emotional exercise with scrapbooks, pictures, postcards, and mementos, and cue up some sad music. After all, you use music to create an environment and set a mood for exercising your body at the gym, so why not do the same for the emotional exercise of your grief? I like to ask patients, on a scale of 1 to 10 with 10 being the highest, "How much grief energy have you stored over the course of your lifetime and how much have you released?" A vast majority tell me that they have stored significantly more grief energy than they have released. I hasten to remind them that their grief is a natural representation of their innermost self. Without it, they can't be whole.

THE LUNG SPIRIT'S COURAGE

The Cowardly Lion in *The Wizard of Oz* was a well-chosen character, intended to make us all feel a little bit better about facing the
demons within our mortal selves. After all, we've been led to believe that big boys and big girls don't cry. For us, courage is seen as
a power that only some people are blessed with. We've been taught
to perceive grief as weakness and courage as strength. As with all
things, the ancient Chinese understood that all dualities were as
one. The thought of being both weak and strong at the same time
is unfathomable for us, but grief is a potentially destructive force
within us that can also germinate our creational energy of courage.

It's impossible to know true courage without experiencing grief.
One of my former Chinese teachers, a centenarian, once explained
to our class that, during the Second Sino-Japanese War, many Chinese families had to leave their homes and dig out living quarters
into the surrounding hills and caves for their safety and survival.
He explained that there was much suffering and grief, especially
among the elderly. He pointed out that when confronted by the
invading Japanese, it was often those with the greatest suffering
and grief who sprang forth to show the most bravery and courage.

They believed that the spirit of the lungs was represented by the
mortal soul. Our mortal soul reflects who we truly are and all we
came to do. It symbolizes the most complete self that we can find
the courage to live through. The mortal soul represents the greatest human potential fully realized—emboldened by the courage to
live out our uncompromised truth—kissed by the tears of our own
grief.

THE KIDNEY SPIRIT'S FEAR

The kidneys are the root organs of the Five Elements Principle.
They represent the water element that's in charge of controlling the

fire element. When the water element is in balance, the fire element is also in balance. If our water element is deficient, our fire is free to run wild. The same fire that warms the house and cooks the food can burn down the house. It can also work the other way. If our water element is excessive, it can put out our fire, leaving us with no means to cook our food or warm our home. In terms of spirit emotions, if our fear is deficient, it can result in joy that becomes uncontrollable mania. Likewise, if our fear is excessive, it can extinguish our heart's joy.

The kidneys hold the key to the spirit's emotion gate, as their fear has governance over all other emotions. For example, many people who suffer from chronic anxiety don't realize that the principal emotion that lies at the root of their stubborn imbalance is actually fear of grief. It's not the anxiety—it's the fearful obsession to control their overwhelming sadness. The depth of repressed grief often drives us to create a compelling thought distraction called "anxiety."

I recently saw a seventy-two-year-old woman who had suffered with generalized anxiety most of her life. Her family expressed growing concerns about what appeared to be an accompanying obsessive-compulsive thought disorder. Her thoughts swirled about over every little inconsequential thing imaginable—she seemed to have lost her mind's "off" switch.

After extensive evaluation, I discovered that she was carrying some very deep emotional wounds from her past. She told me that she was deeply disturbed about living such a disrupted life in a bad marriage. She discovered too late that the man she'd married decades earlier was a substance abuser. She explained to me that she couldn't bring herself to leave him, and that she's carried a deep sadness and regret that her life had been so wasted. She admitted that she had great fear and apprehension about looking at her grief. After a lifetime of repression, her grief had become a tidal wave. I gently and assuredly encouraged her to let go of the fear she had of her grief. Crippling fear held the key to the emotional gates of her other corresponding emotions. This is what forced her to create mental distraction from pain through obsessive thought addiction.

After some time, she began to feel more comfortable with the notion of releasing her grief, and very soon thereafter she was no longer plagued by anxiety and obsessive thinking. By spiritually accepting and releasing her pain, she drained all the energy out of her anxious, obsessive thoughts. By balancing her kidneys' spirit of fear, she was at last able to begin establishing a healing calm in her life.

THE KIDNEY SPIRIT'S CALM

Whenever we think of water, we instinctively think of reflection. When water is calm, it renders greater reflection. In the Five Elements tradition, everything works both ways—calm and reflection are synonymous terms. When there is great calm, there is greater reflection—when there is great reflection, there is greater calm.

Look at the world around you. All you'll see are fast-rushing, turbulent waters, offering little or no reflection. Look at the heavenly reflection of the multiverse above you—on a clear night, your mind is invited to swim in an infinite sea of luminescence. Stargazing has a profound calming effect. Finally, look at the multiverse within you and, as you do so, remember that which manifests externally is equally manifested internally. Every time you go within, you are invited into the sea of your own micromultiverse. There, you can also gaze at the infinite within in order to generate calm. Access to our calming reflection within is provided only by our fearless willingness to look upon our own deepest manifestation of self.

The ancients tell us that the kidney spirit is occupied by the

Will—and our will represents the one force that, if engaged, can determine our destiny. A will afflicted by fear, however, is like a fire extinguished by water. The kidney spirit presents us with a simple formula for spirit balancing. Deep reflection cultivates a spirit of calm that allows the fire of our will to reach our highest destiny.

One of my master teachers once taught me a Qigong exercise that was part of his family tradition for over 3,400 years. The name of the exercise is Building the Mountain of Spiritual Marriage. It needs no further explanation, as its name clearly states its intention. It reminds us that we've all come into consciousness to meet, consummate with, and ultimately emanate as one, from our spirits. As with all relationships, it's a gradual process that must progress in stages. First we discover our true nature, then we unify with it, ultimately becoming one with it. Over time, we add layers to the building of our spiritual mountain. The kidneys lie at the base of the spiritual mountain. By balancing our kidney spirit emotions of fear and calm, we establish a foundation from which to layer our spiritual mountain ever upward.

The Five-Element Organ Spirits (Emotion Blockages)

1. The Liver spirit (Hun)— "The Immortal Soul" (anger)
2. The Heart spirit (Shen)—"The Emperor" (hatred)
3. The Spleen spirit (Shi)—"The Intellect" (anxiety)
4. The Lung spirit (Po)—"The Mortal Soul" (grief)
5. The Kidney spirit (Zhi)—"The Will" (fear)

Here again we can see the physical and spiritual intertwined. The Chinese believed that within us are unique animating spirits exuding from each of our major organs. The spirit within each organ can only be awakened by clearing the emotional blockages. Only by energy balancing can one awaken the powerful visceral spirit energies.

WAKING UP THE ORGAN SPIRITS

Waking up the Liver's Spirit

The liver's spirit was said to be our immortal soul—the internal core of our spiritual self that, throughout our many incarnations, continues to define our core nature, the very way we live, and our unique way of being. In context with the Five Elements, it was believed that the liver's spirit can become blocked when imbalanced by anger.

1. Liver 1 "The Great Esteem Wood"

   This point will assist you with your spiritual growth as well as your confidence, boldness, strength, and purpose. Begin waking up your liver's spirit by simply pressing a finger into the Liver 1 acupuncture point for no more than one minute. As you do, remember to mentally focus on all of the aspects of your life that the liver's spirit is about to help you with.

2. Liver 2 "Walk Between Fire"

   This point will help you with adaptability, flexibility, and being

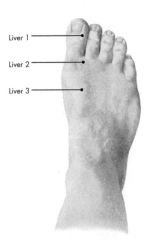

FIGURE 8.2 (a)   *The Liver's Spirit Points*

more open to all forms of love, compassion, and forgiveness. It will also significantly increase your ability to manifest positive visions. Again, press a finger firmly into this point for no more than one minute while focusing on the proper intentions.

3. Liver 3 "Supreme Rushing Earth"

This point will stabilize and root you, as you continue to climb higher in your spiritual ascension. It will also open and stimulate the channels of nourishment from your spirit to the rest of your entire being. Press into this point for one minute with the proper corresponding mental focus.

Waking up the Heart's Spirit

The heart's spirit, or "Shen," was considered the core spirit, and was referred to as The Emperor, as it had the power over all ease and

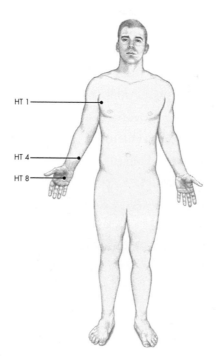

FIGURE 8.2 (b)   The Heart Spirit Points

dis-ease, joy, and hatred, and ultimately physical life and death. The heart's spirit can become blocked by imbalances from hatred.

1. Heart 1 "Utmost Source"
   This point will help you to overcome any self-contempt. It will align you to receive divine love and increase the depth of warmth in all your relationships. Press on this point for one minute and focus the corresponding positive healing intentions.

2. Heart 4 "Spirit Path"
   This point will assist and guide you, keeping you on the proper path of spiritual life. It represents the one true path and enhances your wisdom, discipline, and strength for navigating the straightest course. Press into this point firmly for one minute with the proper focus and attention.

3. Heart 8 "Lesser Palace"
   This point leads one to a fountain of life force that revitalizes beyond anything in the mortal world. It restores, inspires, uplifts, and provides a deep level of internal peace and fulfillment.

Waking up the Spleen's Spirit

The spirit of the spleen governs our intelligence. This spirit rules our ability to concentrate, remember, learn, and to make effectively balanced life decisions. The spleen's spirit can become blocked when imbalanced by anxiety.

1. Spleen 1 "Heaven and Earth Communication"
   This point clears the pathway for better communication between you and all your spirit guidance. It also inspires greater insights and intuitions. Press into this point for one minute with the proper focus.

2. Spleen 3 "Supreme White"
   This is the alignment point for the light body. It increases higher wisdom to help overcome nervous and negative unconscious

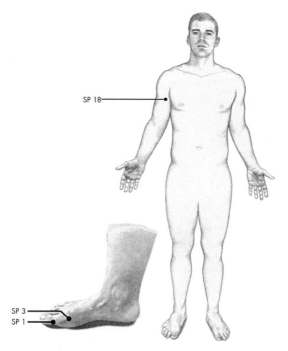

FIGURE 8.2 (c)   *The Spleen Spirit Points*

thought. Press into this point for one minute as you focus your positive intentions accordingly.

3. Spleen 18 "Celestial Stream"

This point will assist with calming the heart and nourishing the spirit. It produces a deep, lasting inner peace. Press into this point while focusing on the proper corresponding healing intention for one minute.

Waking up the Lung's Spirit

The spirit of the lungs reflects the mortal soul. Unlike the immortal soul, this representation of soul and spirit is believed to be given to us anew with each incarnation. This spirit defines our courage to accomplish what we came to do in this lifetime. The lung's spirit can become imbalanced when blocked by grief.

1. Lung 1 "The Central Palace"

   Due to the fact that the lungs have governance over grief, this point is often referred to as the center of the heart. It will help you to overcome grief and heartache, and clear all emotional pathways that block the way of ebullition of spirit. Apply light pressure on this point and focus positive attention for one minute.

2. Lung 2 "Cloud Gate"

   In order for the spirit's higher ch'i to flow, the energy gates must be opened. This point will open the spirit's energy gate, enabling you to receive its abundant healing flow. It will also remove the dark clouds from any old grief that may be in the way. Apply light pressure on this point for one minute while focusing on the desired healing.

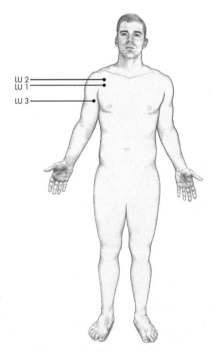

FIGURE 8.2 (d)   The Lung Spirit Points

3. Lung 3 "Heavenly Palace"

This represents the heavenly palace where your spirit will be led. There it will receive abundant joy, protection, and infinite inspiration. Apply light pressure on this point for one minute with the proper intention in mind.

Waking up the Kidney's Spirit

The spirit of the kidneys is where our willpower is rooted. This spirit governs our power to make our life happen through sheer determination. The kidneys' spirit can become blocked when imbalanced by fear.

1. Kidney 1 "Bubbling Spring"

This point will refresh and renew your spirit whenever exhausted. It is a fountain of life to the spirit, especially during times of stress. Apply light pressure on this point for one minute while concentrating on healing intention.

2. Kidney 2 "Blazing Valley"

After the water flows through and refreshes your spirit, it will

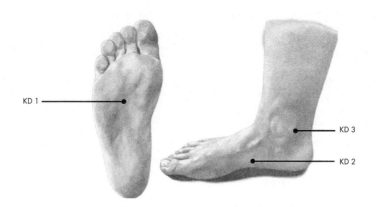

FIGURE 8.2 (e)   The Kidney Spirit Points

then warm and comfort it. This point will produce a soothing and energizing energy to your spirit. Apply light pressure on this point and think about the intended results you desire as you do.

3. Kidney 3 "Greater Mountain Stream Earth"

This point has great force massed from Kidney 1 and 2 that will vibrantly cleanse your spirits of all iniquities, past and present. Apply light pressure on this point for one minute while concentrating on healing intention.

SHEN: THE HEART'S SUPREME SPIRIT

Energy is everywhere, and it is always generating waves that influence every action and every reaction. In the world of energy, everything moves from the subtle internal to the denser external. This is how all things originate—even the emotions that affect our spirits.

According to the ancient Chinese, the energy of dis-ease begins in the spirit of the heart-mind. As the primary residence of the spirit (Shen), they believed that the heart's mind interacts with the soul. These internal references where only the deepest human thoughts and emotions reside represent the innermost rooting place of all disease. Though dis-ease moves its way ever outward from spirit—from heart-mind to physical form—its ripple effect can always be traced from the deepest internal source of our being. They understood well how dis-ease moved from the heart-mind and emotion to the body.

We might think of the internal starting place for dis-ease as the cardiac intrinsic ganglia (heart-mind). Dis-ease first moves from the cardiac intrinsic ganglia to the big brain and body. Negative emotional experiences are first registered in the heart's little brain. They are then simultaneously recorded in the amygdala, hippocampus, central nervous system, and unconscious mind, where they initiate the body's dis-ease process. Once the pattern is established it is then neurologically wired for long-term memory between the amygdala, the hippocampus, and the right prefrontal cortex. The right prefrontal cortex remembers and anticipates. The right brain's remembering can result in depression, and its anticipation can result in anxiety. This was designed by nature to keep us from burning our finger on the stove a second time, but the potential effects of an overzealous right-brain protection system can be devastating to our life-force energy. Whereas the right prefrontal cortex remembers and anticipates, the left prefrontal cortex constructs. Not only is there a positive and negative differential between these two brain hemispheres, the right is more susceptible to being controlled by outside forces, while the left is more inclined to self-empowerment.

The little brain within the heart is where we determine the "good" and the "bad" perceptions of life, as well as the "powerful" and the "powerless" self. Once the message is simultaneously coded into our unconscious mind and body via our nervous system, the message is then wired as a powerful signal that becomes energetically imprinted into our mind/body, affecting our mental and emotional health and immunity. It's in this way that we either become programmed for sympathetic (stress) or parasympathetic (relaxation response) dominance. This is where we either develop a spirit of calm (ease), or a spirit of fear (dis-ease).

SHEN (DIAGNOSTIC)

The first part of this exercise is diagnostic, where practitioner and subject assess in detail all the subject's deep spirit energy blockages. The second part of the exercise is about balancing and healing. In order to clear the Shen, the practitioner must first obtain a Illustrated Shen Clearing Chart (Appendix E). Practitioner and subject must then assume EMT pass/fail position. The practitioner calls out the five negative organ emotions one at a time: anger, hatred, anxiety, grief, and fear. As the practitioner calls out an emotion, they must first record a pass/fail muscle test response. If the

subject's arm drops, this suggests that there is an energy disturbance that corresponds with that emotion. If the arm remains
strong, it indicates that there is no imbalance with that particular
emotion. Next, it is important to pulse test the disturbed emotion
so as to diagnose the degree of imbalance. Pulse test from *negative* 1
to 10. The highest negative numbers represent the greatest disturbances. For example, if anger produces a failed pulse test response at
a range of negative 1 to 3, it is only minor. If it fails at a negative 4
to 6 pulse, it is moderate. A negative 7 to 10 pulse test response,
however, should be considered severe.

Next, the Internal Root reference should be tested. This reveals
the source or sources of the subject's negative emotional energy
blockages. There are six potential sources in all, which are: mother,
father, natal family, married family, culture, and world. When our
unconscious mind stores negative emotional life experiences, it catalogs them in neurological compartments in the brain. Each stored
negative energy is directly associated with one of these five Internal
Root References. Before testing for the Internal Root References,
practitioners must make sure to explain to all subjects exactly what
they are about to do. Painful emotions may surface during this
juncture of the exercise. These emotions may represent a potential
healing crisis that some may not be ready to contend with.

Once the practitioner feels ready to proceed, they should note
the present age of the subject by drawing a line just beneath the
corresponding number on the Ages of Shen Blockages section of
their Shen Clearing Chart. Then, they should once again prepare
to assume proper EMT pass/fail posture with their subject. First,
the practitioner should call out "Prebirth." This will reveal any Shen
blockages that might have occurred while in the womb. Now, the
practitioner will call out the remaining ages, one at a time, beginning with "One," and so on. If, when audibly calling out any age, the
subject's arm falls, the practitioner should circle it on the chart. At
each age, the practitioner must call out the negative emotion that

failed above when tested. Finally the subject's emotional blockages that correspond with the age that has failed must be pulse tested from a negative 1 to 10. So, if the subject's arm dropped at age of three, and their earlier test failed with grief, then it is important to pulse test the degree of grief that the subject is holding on to.

CLEARING THE SHEN (SPIRIT BALANCING)

The balancing healing part of the Shen Clearing protocol is very simple. The practitioner and subject interface in the standing pass/fail position. The practitioner must ask the subject to close their eyes. The practitioner must then recite the following speech, or a similar monologue, to the subject:

"Now I will ask you to exhale, releasing a cleansing breath from exactly where your breath is, followed by a deep inhale breath. Hold the breath in for a count of three . . . one, two, and three . . . then release the breath fully, holding it out for a count of three . . . one, two, and three. Once again, take another deep breath, filling your lungs to full capacity. Now, again, hold the breath in for a full count of three . . . one, two, and three. Again, fully release the breath and hold the breath out for a count of three . . . one, two, and three. Finally, take your third and final deep inhale. Hold the breath in for a count of three . . . one, two, and three. Now, while still holding the breath in, I will ask you to open your mouth and pause for a slow count of three . . . one, two and three. Now fully release the breath.

"Keeping your eyes closed, I will now ask you to draw upon your highest, deepest intentions to profoundly heal your life. You have carried deep destabilizing energies within your heart-mind and spirit for far too long. You will now draw up from within you the highest power of love and innermost determination to release and let go of all the imbalanced energies that have, up until now, attached to your spirit. This is your touchstone moment. You are about to transform and heal your entire being. I will ask you to simply release all the energy blockages that we've just discovered together. Regardless of the what, where, why, when, and how, these blockages are merely energies that you have the complete power to release, and you will." (Practitioners should now briefly and swiftly summarize the subject's specific blockages about to be released, instructing the subject to release each one.)

Finally, to demonstrate the healing that just took place, the practitioner must once gain call out the previously discovered blockages while testing the muscle strength of the subject. You will find a very strong response this time, indicating the energy clearance. Ask how long the clearance will last and muscle test the responses for one day, one week, one month, one year, ten years, 100 years, an eternity. It always results in eternal clearance.

CLEARING THE SHEN WITH HEART FIRE

The word *atavism* refers to a resurfacing of a characteristic in an organism after generations of being absent. Atavisms are genetic mechanisms. They suggest that, no matter how hard we may try to escape our inherited characteristics, they are at some level bound and destined to surface through our map of mechanisms. I believe emotions are atavistic in the sense that they represent tendencies from our gene map, tendencies that are likely to surface and resurface over and over.

The most disabling of all blockages to the human spirit are those negative emotional tendencies that haunt us unceasingly. They seem to be a reflection of our core self—a part of who we are. In order for us to transcend our emotional atavisms, we must channel their core energy through the most powerful energy incinerator that we have—our heart fire. Before we do so, we must first empower our heart fire by accepting full responsibility for the blockage.

Many mistakenly insist on blaming their deepest, indelible emotional perturbations on some "other." All emotional disturbances become channeled by our atavistic tendencies into the storehouse of the unconscious mind. There, they take control over us as we infuse them with emotion, neurology, and repetition. The power of the emotional atavism lies within the unconscious mind. The limiting blockages that were likely triggered by people, places, and things beyond our control end up becoming our unconscious, self-limiting blockages. It is only due to our own unconscious repetition and neuroemotional infusion that they grow into spirit-disabling monsters in our minds.

As the literal translation suggests, atavisms are mechanistic. Our deepest emotional disturbances make connections with our cells, molecules, and DNA. To invoke healing through such a complex matrix, we must reach beyond our material mechanisms into the atomic and subatomic realms of our most powerful energy field. We must trump the power of the brain and its connection to the subconscious mind.

The heart generates five times more electrical energy than the brain, and sixty times more electromagnetic energy than the brain. Every single one of our 100 trillion cells is energetically aligned with the heart's electromagnetic field. Where the negative emotional brain (amygdala/hippocampus/right prefrontal cortex) is wired to the unconscious mind, the positive emotional brain (left prefrontal cortex) is wired to the superconscious mind. The positive emotional brain and superconscious mind are where the heart fire is generated. The heart fire represents our miracle potential. Only through the heart fire can we burn away our deepest emotional disturbances.

Ironically, many people get nervous at the suggestion that they can delete a negative, lifelong emotional stigma. They often discover a distorted attachment to the very emotion they are most desperate to cleanse. This reveals the power of emotional atavisms.

Though negative, they become familiar spirits. For some, they may be the only remaining attachment to very powerful memories. Emotional atavisms often find ways to attach to those people, places, and things that generate the most compelling energy in our negative emotional brain and unconscious mind. They may drain us of our power, but they generate a compelling force.

Clearing the Shen with Heart Fire can be performed without the assistance of a practitioner. As with all Whole Health energy healing protocols, begin this exercise by ensuring that you will have undisturbed quiet for a good fifteen minutes or so. Then, exactly like the HeartMath heart entrainment exercise, you must begin by taking three deep breaths, and envisioning them as being drawn into the heart rather than the lungs. With eyes closed and both hands placed open and over the heart, visualize a fire of white healing light blazing in your heart. This is the healing flame that burns off any negative blockages that may stand in the way of the spirit's highest possible ascension to a state of pure joy. Take a few moments to build and empower the healing fire. Now picture yourself drawing all past emotional disturbances in the fire. It is not necessary to recall any specific incidents. As with most energy-healing protocols, it is more about the power of intention than it is about any details or recalling of events. Take several minutes to feed your fire with only two key intentions in mind.

Your first primary intention is to be determined to burn off any and all energies that block your spirit from joy. The second is to impose an intention of closure. You must be determined to finish what you've set out to do. When tapped into with sufficient focus and concentration, your superconscious mind has more than enough power to clear your Shen from these blockages permanently. When it comes to any healing release, you must believe in your power of closure!

Continue for several minutes and then gently open your eyes. Keep your mind quiet and clear for another few moments as you gradually move back into the flow of your day. As you do so, know that you have permanently cleared your spirit of any blockages to attaining joy. Also, keep in mind that while you may have cleared past blockages, you will have to keep up with day-to-day emotional accumulations. Therefore, it is important to practice Clear the Shen with Heart Fire at least once a month.

MERGING SHEN WITH WOOD

The main purpose of balancing one's energy is to heal the body, mind, and spirit. The key to healing the spirit is increasing the internal energy. The simplest exercise for increasing the internal energy and instantly bringing calm to the spirit is by Merging Shen with Wood. Gently place the tip of both your middle fingers (Pericardium 9) on the neck just behind and below both ears (Gallbladder 20). Bow your head slightly and leave the fingers there in place for three minutes. Close your eyes and envision yourself transmit-

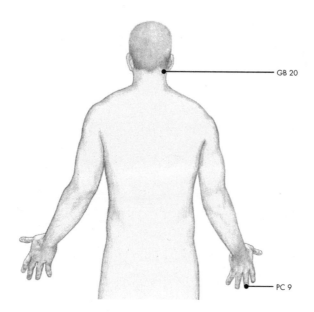

FIGURE 8.3   Merging Shen with Wood

ting healing energy to your innermost spirit and mind. This will increase the flow of energy to your internal being, gently uplifting your spirit energy and bringing you peace.

MAINTAINING SHEN CLARITY

Once the Shen blockages from the past are cleared, it is important to keep one's spirit clear moving forward. We must remember that energy is accumulative, and that we are both conduits *and* collectors of energy. With every passing day we encounter potentially powerful life-changing experiences. Such experiences are capable of initiating new patterns of dis-ease that create Shen blockages. Whole Health has developed brain reprogramming, mind-changing systems for keeping the Shen clear as you move forward.

The spirit can only be kept clear if the energy that is presented to the cardiac intrinsic ganglia is positive. To keep clear, one has to remain positive. The signal from the heart's little brain to the amygdale, hippocampus, central nervous system, and unconscious mind has to be recorded as a positive entrainment signal in order for the spirit to remain unblocked.

EPILOGUE

We now find ourselves caught in the crosscurrent between old and new paradigms. Everywhere around and deep within us there is great turbulence. It's as if our new identity was moving forward, even as our former identity was moving backward, and all at warp speed. We are in the midst of an identity crisis of epic proportions. During this time of great metamorphosis, many are finding their unconscious thoughts and emotions increasingly difficult to manage. The stresses associated with such a transformational shift continue to bring great pressure to bear on our most subtle, internal intricacies. The transmutations within our deepest thoughts and emotions are also producing radical changes regarding our deeper needs. Much of that which nurtured and healed us a mere decade ago simply no longer can.

Everything is reforming—everything—including who we are, how we are, and how we heal, as the current health care system struggles to facilitate the kind of body, mind, and spirit wholeness we now require.

As our consciousness expands, we are becoming increasingly more sensitive. Our evolving sensitivities demand new strategies to support our nurturance and healing in ways more attuned to our changing needs. And while new systems to meet our deeper needs are evolving, we continue to wade through the powerful crosscurrent of shifting paradigms. Our transformational growth is thrusting forward even as our most fundamental systems continue to lag behind. This is especially true in the food and health care industries.

Today, our foods are genetically modified—fat, sugar, pesticide, and additive-laden beyond recognition. Up to 80 percent of the prepackaged foods on our grocery shelves are banned in most other countries. Many of our most common foods contain extremely toxic, carcinogenic chemicals like bisphenol A, bromates, phthalates, bovine growth hormone, and vinyl chloride. In fact, much of our food is now so denatured that it actually has the power to cause and/or mimic disease. Our medicines are even more harmful.

Our current health care establishment is still driven by a pharmaceutical model that insists on producing remedies so noxious that they are often far worse than the conditions they are prescribed for. You can learn everything you need to know about the disturbing truth regarding our medicines by simply listening to the side effects and contraindications narrative at the conclusion of any pharmaceutical television commercial. Once the solution to our ills, our food and medicine have now become the problem. Thankfully, the fading toxic food and medicine paradigm is gradually giving way to a new holistic archetype.

When biotech pioneer Leroy Hood first coined the term *P4 medicine* shortly after the turn of the new millennium, the new paradigm in health care was born. P4 is a revolutionary concept that stands for predictive, preventive, personalized, and participatory medicine. Unlike the fading health care paradigm, where the system sought to manage the patient's disease, P4 medicine focuses on the patient's management of their own health through diet, nutritional supplementation, exercise, and mind/body strategies.

Whole Health is an energy-based, P4 holistic health care system for the twenty-first century. Its aim is to educate, inspire, and empower individuals to administer their own health care with safe, effective, time-tested strategies. Its primary healing agents are clean, natural foods, nutritional supplements, and energy medicine protocols. Its strategy is based on personalized, participatory disease prevention, with a focus on tuning into the causal roots of disease patterns. *Whole Health* empowers its readers with a "how-to" participatory approach to holistic nutrition and energy medicine.

The Whole Health Healing System is the culmination of my three decades of dedication to the art of natural healing. It is my heartfelt intention to gift all that I have learned through the vehicles of this book and system, for which it is named, to an ever-deserving world.

APPENDIX A
Whole Health Materia Medica Index

ACIDOSIS

World Organics Triple Strength Chlorophyll (100 mg capsules):
2 capsules 3 times per day with water on empty stomach

Baking soda: ½ teaspoon in 3 ounces water before bed

Natural Calm Magnesium Citrate Powder: 1 teaspoon in 4 ounces
water before bed

ADD/ADHD

Nordic Naturals DHA (500 mg capsules): 1 capsule 2 times per
day on empty stomach

Vitamin D (1,500 units, capsules): 2 capsules per day on empty
stomach

Solgar VM 75 Multivitamin: 1 with breakfast

Protein at breakfast

Increase egg whites, fish, and beans in the diet

Test for food reactions

ADDISON'S DISEASE

Pantothenic Acid (500 mg tablets): 1 tablet 3 times per day
with food

New Chapter Holy Basil (800 mg capsules): 1 capsule 3 times per
day on empty stomach

Homeopathic Nux Vomica (pellets 30c potency): dissolve
3 pellets under tongue 3 times per day on empty stomach

Bach Flower Remedies Hornbeam (drops): dissolve 3 drops in
3 ounces water 3 times per day on empty stomach

ALLERGIES (SEASONAL)

BioAllers Allergy Tincture (drops): dissolve 10 drops under
tongue 3 times per day on empty stomach

Quercetin (500 mg tablets): 1 tablet 3 times per day with food

Vitamin C Complex (1,000 mg tablets): 2 tablets with meals—6 total

Test for food reactions

ALZHEIMER'S DISEASE

EGCG Max brand epigallicatechin gallate (700 mg capsules): 3 capsules per day on empty stomach

Nordic Naturals DHA (450 mg capsules): 3 capsules per day on empty stomach

Vinpocetine (10 mg capsules): 2 capsules per day on empty stomach

ANEMIA

Methyl B_{12} (1,000 mcg chewable tablet): 1 tablet per day with food

Dessicated Liver Tabs (700 mg tablets): 6 tablets per day with food

Yellow Dock Root Tea: 2 cups per day

Liquid Chlorophyll: 2 tablespoons in 6 ounces water 3 times daily

ANGINA

Jarrow Formulas Q Absorb (200 mg capsules): 2 capsules per day on empty stomach

Jarrow Formulas Ribose (powder): 2 scoops in water per day on empty stomach

Natural Calm Magnesium Citrate (powder): 2 teaspoons per day in water

Nordic Naturals Omega 3 Fish Oil (1,000 mg capsules): 2 capsules per day with food

ANTIBIOTICS

Oreganol (drops): 10 drops 3 times per day after meals

Goldenseal (tincture): 25 drops 3 times per day on empty stomach

Monolaurin (600 mg capsules): 4 capsules per day on empty
    stomach

Colloidal Silver (drops): 6 drops 3 times per day on empty
    stomach

ANTI-INFLAMMATORIES

Zyflamend (capsules): 4 capsules per day on empty stomach

Wobenzyme (capsules): 4 capsules per day on empty stomach

Nordic Naturals Omega 3 Fish Oil (1,000 mg capsules): 3 capsules
    per day with food

Turmeric: to spice food

Rosemary Tea: 2 cups per day

ANTIMETASTATIC

(See Cancer)

ANXIETY

Kava Kava (herbal tincture): 25 drops 3 times per day on empty
    stomach

Passion Flower (500 mg capsules): 4 capsules per day on empty
    stomach

L-Theanine (100 mg capsules): 3 capsules per day on empty
    stomach

Natural Calm Magnesium Citrate (powder): 1 teaspoon in
    4 ounces water before bed

AROMATASE INHIBITORS (INHIBIT
CANCER-CAUSING ESTROGENS)

ReserveAge Resveratrol (500 mg capsules): 1 capsule per day with
    food

Now brand Indole 3-carbinol (200 mg capsules): 3 capsules per
    day on empty stomach

Physician's Formula Chrysin (500 mg capsules): 4 capsules per day
on empty stomach

ARTERIOSCLEROSIS

Serrapeptase (40,000 units, capsules): 2 capsules per day on empty
stomach

Jarrow Formulas MK-7 (90 mcg—capsules): 3 capsules per day on
empty stomach

Lewis Labs Lecithin Granules: 3 tablespoons per day in beverage

ARTHRITIS

Country Life MSM/GS Complex (tablets): 3 tablets per day on
empty stomach

Vitamin D (1,500 units, capsules): 2 capsules per day on empty
stomach

Bromelain (500 mg capsules): 2 capsules midmorning and
2 capsules midafternoon on empty stomach

Homeopathic Bryonia Alba (pellets, 6X potency): dissolve
3 pellets under tongue 3 times per day on empty stomach

ASTHMA

L-Cysteine (500 mg capsules): 2 capsules per day on empty
stomach

Lobelia (tincture): dissolve 25 drops in 3 ounces water 3 times
per day on empty stomach

Marshmallow Root (500 mg capsules): 2 capsules on empty
stomach twice per day

Mullein Tea: 2 cups per day

ATRIAL FIBRILLATION (IRREGULAR HEARTBEAT)

Magnesium Taurate (125 mg capsules): 4 capsules per day with
food

Natural Calm Magnesium Citrate: 1 teaspoon in 4 ounces water
before bed

Ashwagandha (450 mg capsules): 3 capsules per day on empty
stomach

Planetary Herbs Triphala (500 mg capsules): 3 capsules per day on
empty stomach

Jarrow Formulas Q Absorb (capsules): 2 capsules per day on
empty stomach

Nordic Naturals Omega 3 Fish Oil (1,000 mg capsules): 2 capsules
2 times per day with food

Now Grape Seed Extract (60 mg capsules): 2 capsules 2 times per
day on empty stomach

AUTISM

Cilantro (tincture): 25 drops in 3 ounces water 3 times per day
on empty stomach

L-Carnosine (500 mg capsules): 2 capsules per day on empty
stomach

Vitamin D (1,500 mg capsules): 2 capsules per day with food

Vitamin B_{12} Methylcobalamin (pellets): 5,000 mcg per day with
food

Anti-*Candida* diet

Dairy-free diet

Gluten-free diet

BLADDER (URINARY TRACT INFECTIONS)

Cranberry (500 mg capsules): 2 capsules twice per day on empty
stomach

Homeopathic *Eupatorium Purpureum* (pellets, 6X potency):
dissolve 3 pellets under tongue 3 times per day on
empty stomach

Homeopathic Cantharis (pellets, 6X potency): dissolve 3 pellets
under tongue 3 times per day on empty stomach

Vitamin C Complex (1,000 mg tablets): 2 tablets every 2 hours
(total of 10,000 mg)

BLEPHARITIS

Homeopathic Cantharis (pellets, 6X potency): dissolve 3 pellets
under tongue 3 times per day on empty stomach
Carno-See (drops): as directed
Colloidal Silver (drops): dissolve 2 drops in each eye 2 times
per day

BLOOD BUILDERS

(See Anemia)

BLOOD PRESSURE (HIGH)

Dr. Michael Murray's ACE Peptide (500 mg capsules): 3 capsules
per day on empty stomach
Folic Acid (400 mcg capsules): 3 per day with food
Hawthorn Berry (tincture): dissolve 25 drops in 3 ounces water
3 times per day on empty stomach
Magnesium Taurate (125 mg capsules): 4 per day with food
Now Grape Seed Extract (60 mg capsules): 4 capsules per day
on empty stomach
Celery Root (tincture, with 3nB): dissolve 25 drops in 3 ounces
water 3 times per day on empty stomach

BLOOD PRESSURE (LOW)

Celtic Sea Salt: a pinch with each major meal
Indian Spikenard (tincture): dissolve 25 drops in 3 ounces water
3 times per day
Vitamin E (Gamma) (400 units, capsules): 3 capsules per day with
food
Korean Ginseng Tea: 2 cups per day

BLOOD SUGAR (HIGH)

Cinnamon (500 mg capsules): 4 capsules per day on empty stomach
Bitter Melon Tea: 2 cups per day

BLOOD SUGAR (LOW)

Solgar Chromium GTF (200 mcg capsules): 1 capsule after meals
L-Glutamine (500 mg capsules): 1 capsule midmorning and
    1 midafternoon on empty stomach
B 50 Complex (tablets): 1 capsule with each major meal—3 total
    per day
Zinc Chelate (25 mg tablets): 1 tablet per day with food

BLOOD THINNERS

(See Anti-Inflammatories)

BONE HEALTH

Garden of Life Bone Grow System: as directed
Jarrow Formulas Jarrowsil (drops): dissolve 6 drops in water
    3 times per day after meals
World Organics Triple Strength Chlorophyll (100 mg capsules):
    3 capsules per day on empty stomach

BREAST TENDERNESS (PREMENSTRUAL)

Evening Primrose Oil (300 mg capsules): 1 per day on empty
    stomach
Chasteberry Herb (tincture): dissolve 25 drops in 3 ounces water
    3 times per day on empty stomach
Raspberry Leaf Tea: 2 cups per day
Calendula Oil: as needed for topical rub

BRONCHITIS

N-Acetyl-Cysteine (500 mg capsules): 2 per day on empty
 stomach

Myrrh (tincture): dissolve 25 drops in 3 ounces water 3 times per
 day on empty stomach

Mullein Tea: 2 cups per day

Homeopathic *Thuja Occidentalis* (pellets, 6X potency): dissolve
 3 pellets under tongue 3 times per day on empty stomach

CALCIUM

(The three most absorbable—choose one):

Garden of Life Bone Grow System: as directed on label

BioCalth (300 mg capsules): 1 capsule 3 times per day on empty
 stomach

Advacal (500 mg capsules): 2 per day on empty stomach

CALCIUM DEPOSITS: (SPURS, STONES, AND PLAQUES)

Serrapeptase (40,000 units, capsules): 1 capsule twice daily on
 empty stomach

Bromelain (500 mg capsules): 1 capsule twice daily on empty
 stomach

Jarrow MK-7 (90 mcg capsules): 2 capsules per day on empty
 stomach

Lewis Labs Lecithin Granules: 3 tablespoons per day in beverage

CANCER

Sugar-free diet

Fermentation-free diet

Avoid yeast, vinegar, nuts, melons, mushrooms, aged cheeses,
 beer, wine, and champagne

World Organics Triple Strength Chlorophyll (100 mg capsules):
 2 capsules 3 times per day on empty stomach

Baking soda: ½ teaspoon in 3 ounces water before bed

Nature's Sunshine Cell Reg (Paw Paw Herb) (12.5 mg capsules):
1 capsule per day with food

Lemongrass Tea: 2 cups per day

Jarrow Formulas IP6 (Inositol Hexaphosphate) (615 mg capsules):
2 capsules per day with food

Amazing Herbs Black Cumin Seed Oil (500 mg capsules):
4 capsules per day on empty stomach

Turmeric: spice with food

ProFibe Fruit Pectin Powder: 2 scoops in beverage per day on
empty stomach

Cardiovascular Research Ellagic Acid (500 mg capsules):
2 capsules per day on empty stomach

Planetary Herbals Triphala (500 mg capsules): 2 capsules per day
on empty stomach

CANDIDIASIS

Solgar Caprylic Acid (tablets): 1 tablet with meals—3 total

Pau D'arco (capsules): 2 capsules 2 times per day on empty
stomach

Jarrow Formulas EPS (capsules): 2 capsules 2 times per day on
empty stomach

Grapefruit Seed Extract (drops): dissolve 6 drops in 3 ounces
water 3 times per day with food

Avoid all processed sugars and fermented foods

CATARACTS

L-Carnosine (500 mg tablets): 4 tablets per day on empty
stomach

Carno-See (drops): as directed

Vitamin D (1,500 units, capsules): 2 capsules per day on empty
stomach

CHOLESTEROL

Jarrow Formulas GPLC (Glyco-Carnitine) (500 mg capsules): 2 capsules per day on empty stomach

Jarrow Formulas Pantethine (450 mg): 3 per day with food

Garlicin 4000 (capsules): 1 capsule per day on empty stomach

Red Rice Yeast (500 mg capsules): 2 capsules per day on empty stomach

Nordic Naturals Omega 3 Fish Oil (1,000 mg capsules): 2 capsules 3 times per day with food

CIRCULATION

Vitamin E (Gamma) (400 units, capsules): 2 capsules per day with food

Lewis Labs Lecithin Granules: 3 tablespoons per day in beverage

Now Grape Seed Extract (60 mg capsules): 3 capsules per day on empty stomach

COLD AND FLU

(See Virus)

COLD SORES

L-Lysine Ointment: applied topically as directed

L-Lysine (1,000 mg tablets): 1 tablet 2 times per day on empty stomach

Lemon Balm (tincture): dissolve 25 drops in 3 ounces water 3 times per day on empty stomach

Ecological Formulas Monolaurin (600 mg capsules): 2 capsules with meals—4 total per day

COLIC

Homeopathic Pulsatilla (pellets, 6X potency): crush and dissolve 2 pellets in warm water and take 2 times per day on empty stomach

Avoid dairy, and drink soy/substitute Meyenberg's Goat's Milk
Formula, or Biotics Nutri-Clear Rice Formula

COLITIS

Jarrow Formulas EPS (Probiotics) (capsules): 2 capsules per day on
empty stomach

Nature Most Multi Enzyme (tablets): 1 tablet with breakfast and
1 tablet with lunch

Folic Acid (400 mcg tablets): 2 tablets per day with food

B_{12} (Methylcobalamin) (1,000 mg tablets): 2 tablets per day with
food

Homeopathic Ipecac (pellets, 30X potency): dissolve 3 pellets
under tongue 3 times per day on empty stomach

CONSTIPATION

Natural Calm Magnesium Citrate (powder): 1 teaspoon in
4 ounces water before bed

Atri Aloe V (465 mgs tablets): 1 before bed

Flaxseed Husks (ground): 2 tablespoons per day with
food

COUGH

Wintergreen Tea: 2 cups per day

Myrrh (tincture): 25 drops in 3 ounces water 3 times per day on
empty stomach

Wild Cherry Bark (syrup): as directed

Mullein (tincture): dissolve 25 drops in 3 ounces water 3 times per
day on empty stomach

CRAMPS

Cramp Bark Herb (tincture): dissolve 25 drops in 3 ounces water
3 times per day on empty stomach

Raspberry Leaf Tea: 1 cup

White Willow Bark Tea: 1 cup

Homeopathic Hypericum (pellets, 30c potency): dissolve 3 pellets
   under tongue 3 times per day on empty stomach

CRAVINGS (SUGAR AND STARCH)

Chromium (200 mcg tablets): 1 tablet with meals—3 total

Carbs Away (tablets): 1 tablet with meals—3 total

L-Glutamine (500 mg tablets): 1 tablet midmorning and 1 tablet
   midafternoon on empty stomach

C-REACTIVE PROTEIN (ELEVATED)

Serrapeptase (20,000 units, tablets): 3 tablets per day on empty
   stomach

Bromelain (500 mg tablets): 3 tablets per day on empty stomach

B_{12} (Methylcobalamin) (5,000 mcg tablets): 1 tablet per day with
   food

Folic Acid (400 mcg tablets): 3 tablets per day with food

Trimethylglycine (500 mg tablets): 2 tablets per day with food

CROHN'S DISEASE

(See Colitis)

DANDRUFF

Nordic Naturals Cod Liver Oil: 1 tablespoon 3 times per day with
   food

Wash hair with PSO Medis Shampoo

DEMENTIA

DHA (500 mg capsules): 2 capsules per day on empty stomach

Vinpocetine (10 mg tablets): 2 tablets per day on empty stomach

EGCE Max (700 mg capsules): 2 capsules per day on empty
   stomach

DEPRESSION

St. John's Wort with 5 percent Hyperforin (200 mg capsules):
   3 capsules per day on empty stomach
5 HTP (500 mg capsules): 2 capsules per day on empty stomach
Tulsi Tea: 2 cups per day
Holy Basil (800 mg capsules): 2 capsules per day on empty
   stomach

DERMATITIS

Homeopathic Sulphur (pellets, 6X potency): dissolve 3 pellets
   under tongue 3 times per day on empty stomach
ReserveAge Collagen Resveratrol (tablets): 2 tablets per day with
   food
Zinc Gluconate (50 mg tablets): 1 tablet per day with food
Alpha Lipoic Acid (50 mg tablets): 2 tablets per day on empty
   stomach
Test for food reactions

DIABETES

(See Blood Sugar, High)

DIARRHEA

Homeopathic Colocynthis (pellets, 6X potency): dissolve 3 pellets
   under tongue 3 times per day on empty stomach
Jarrow Formulas EPS (capsules): 2 capsules per day on empty
   stomach
Diet of white rice and applesauce

DIGESTION (POOR)

Nature Most Multi Enzymes (tablets): 1 tablet with breakfast and
   lunch

Biotics Nutri-Clear (meal replacement): 1 shake made with rice
    milk at breakfast
Homeopathic Carbo Veg (pellets, 6X potency): dissolve 3 pellets
    under tongue 3 times per day on empty stomach
Test for food reactions

DIVERTICULITIS/DIVERTICULOSIS

Aloe Vera Juice: drink 3 ounces 3 times per day before meals
Jarrow EPS (capsules): 3 capsules per day on empty stomach
Nature Most Multi Enzymes (tablets): 1 tablet with meals—
    3 total
Test for food reactions

DOWN SYNDROME

Selenium (100 mcg tablets): 1 tablet per day with food
Pycnogenol (50 mg capsules): 2 capsules per day on empty
    stomach
Chewable Zinc (10 mg tablets): 1 tablet per day with food
Nordic Naturals Flavored DHA (liquid): as directed
Jarrow Formulas Q Absorb (200 mgs capsules): 1 capsule per day
    with food

DYSPEPSIA (ACID STOMACH)

Chewable Papain tablets: 1 tablet with breakfast and 1 tablet with
    lunch
Homeopathic Robinia pellets (6X potency): dissolve 3 pellets
    under tongue 3 times per day on empty stomach
(Also see Acidosis)

EAR INFECTION

Colloidal Silver (drops applied in ear): put 4 drops in ear 3 times
    per day

Oreganol Oil (drops): 6 drops added to food or beverage 3 times per day

Vitamin C Complex (tablets/chewable for children): adults 5,000 mg per day/children under 12—500 mg per day

ECZEMA

Burdock Root (tincture): dissolve 25 drops in 3 ounces water 3 times per day on empty stomach

Nordic Naturals Omega 3 (capsules): 2 capsules 2 times per day with food

Homeopathic Aresnicum (pellets, 6c potency): dissolve 3 pellets under tongue 3 times per day on empty stomach

Test for food reactions

ENDOMETRIOSIS

Vitamin E Gamma (400 mg capsules): 3 capsules per day on empty stomach

Evening Primrose Oil (300 mg capsules): 1 capsule per day with food

DIM (100 mg capsules): 1 capsule per day on empty stomach

Yeast-free, low-sugar diet

EPILEPSY (SEIZURES)

L-Taurine (500 mg capsules): 2 capsules per day on empty stomach

L-Glutamine (powder): 5,000 mgs per day on empty stomach

Magnesium Taurate (125 mg capsules): 3 capsules per day with food

ESTROGEN (DEFICIENCY)

Emerita Transdermal Bio Identical Estrogen (cream): rub ¼ teaspoon on wrists 2 times per day

DIM (100 mg capsules): 1 capsule per day on empty stomach

Spirutein Soy Protein (power shake): 20 grams per day

Evening Primrose Oil (300 mg capsules): 1 capsule per day with food

Increase soy in diet

FAT BURNING (SUPPORT LIPID METABOLISM)

Lewis Labs Lecithin Granules: 3 tablespoons per day in beverage

Jarrow Formulas GPLC (Glyco-Carnitine) (500 mg capsules): 2 capsules per day on empty stomach

Jarrow Pantethine (450 mg capsules): 3 capsules per day with food

Methionine (500 mg capsules): 2 capsules per day on empty stomach

FATIGUE

New Chapter Holy Basil (800 mg capsules): 2 capsules per day on empty stomach

Tulsi Tea: 2 cups per day

Korean Ginseng Tea: 3 cups per day

Solgar Spirulina (750 mg capsules): 3 capsules 3 times per day with food

Jarrow Formulas DMAE (100 mg tablets): 1 tablet 2 times per day with meals

Jarrow Formulas Yum Yum DHA (120 mg chewables): 3 per day with food

FEVER

White Willow Bark Tea: 1 cup 2 to 3 times per day

Wobenzyme (capsules): 2 capsules every 3 hours

Serrapeptase (20,000 units, capsules): 1 capsule 3 times per day

FIBROIDS

Amazing Herbs Black Cumin Seed Oil (500 mg capsules): 2 capsules 2 times per day on empty stomach

Pau D'arco (500 mg capsules): 2 capsules 2 times per day on
  empty stomach
Vitamin E (Gamma) (400 units, capsules): 3 capsules per day on
  empty stomach
Fermentation-free diet

FIBROMYALGIA

Zyflamend (capsules): 2 capsules every 3 hours
Homeopathic Bryonia Alba (pellets, 30c potency): dissolve
  3 pellets under tongue 3 times per day on empty stomach
Nordic Naturals Ultimate Omega with CoQ10 (capsules):
  2 capsules 2 times per day on empty stomach

FLATULENCE

Homeopathic Carbo Veg (pellets, 6X potency): dissolve 3 pellets
  under tongue 3 times per day on empty stomach
Charcoal (125 mg tablets): 1 capsule after meals

GALLSTONES

Jarrow Formulas MK-7 (90 mcg capsules): 2 capsules 2 times per
  day on empty stomach
Serrapeptase (20,000 units, capsules): 1 capsule 3 times per day
  on empty stomach
Lewis Labs Lecithin Granules: 1 tablespoon 3 times per day in
  beverage
Homeopathic Nat Sulph (pellets, 30c potency): dissolve 3 pellets
  under tongue 3 times per day on empty stomach
Quantum Herbs Barberry (tincture): dissolve 25 drops in 3 ounces
  water 3 times per day on empty stomach

GLAUCOMA

Bilberry (100 mg capsules): 2 capsules 3 times per day on empty
  stomach

Source Naturals Zeaxanthin/Lutein Formula (10 mg capsules):
2 capsules 2 times per day on empty stomach

L-Carnosine (500 mg capsules): 2 capsules 2 times per day on
empty stomach

Carno-See (drops): as directed

GOUT

Homeopathic Bryonia Alba (pellets, 6X potency): dissolve
3 pellets under tongue 3 times per day on empty
stomach

Bromelain (500 mg capsules): 2 capsules between meals 2 times
per day on empty stomach

Test for food reactions

Decrease animal proteins

H1N1 SWINE FLU

(See Virus)

HAIR GRAYING (TO PREVENT)

Fo-Ti (1,000 mg capsules): 1 capsule 2 times per day on empty
stomach

Nature's Plus Ultra Hair (tablets): 2 tablets per day with food

HAIR LOSS (TO PREVENT)

Natures Plus Ultra Hair (tablets): 2 tablets per day with food

B 100 Complex (tablets): 1 with meals—3 total

Nature Most Zinc Gluconate (50 mg tablets): 1 tablet per day
with food

HEADACHES

Chrysanthemum Flower Tea: 2 cups per day

White Willow Bark (500 mg capsules): 2 capsules 2 times per day
on empty stomach

Wobenzyme (capsules): 2 capsules every 3 hours on empty
   stomach

HEART HEALTH

Jarrow Formulas Q Absorb (200 mg capsules): 1 capsule per day
   on empty stomach
Jarrow Formulas GPLC (500 mg capsules): 2 capsules per day on
   empty stomach
Cardiovascular Research Magnesium Taurate (125 mg capsules):
   4 per day on empty stomach
Hawthorn Berry (500 mg capsules): 2 capsules 2 times per day
   on empty stomach
Folic Acid (400 mcg capsules): 2 capsules 2 times per day with
   food
Jarrow Formulas Ribose (200 grams, powder): 2 scoops per day

HEAVY METAL TOXICITY

Cilantro (tincture): dissolve 25 drops in 3 ounces water 3 times
   per day on empty stomach
ProFibe Fruit Pectin (powder): 1 scoop in water 2 times per day
   on empty stomach
Homeopathic Mercurius (for Mercury) (pellets, 6X potency):
   dissolve 3 pellets under tongue 1 time per day for 90 days
Homeopathic Plumbum (for lead) (pellets, 6X potency): dissolve
   3 pellets under tongue 1 time per day for 90 days
Homeopathic Alumina (for aluminum) (pellets, 6X potency):
   dissolve 3 pellets under tongue 1 time per day for 90 days

HEMORRHOIDS

Citrus Bioflavonoid (500 mg tablets): 2 tablets 2 times per day
   with food
Homeopathic *Aesculus hippocastanum* (pellets, 6X potency): dissolve
   3 pellets under tongue 3 times per day on empty stomach

HEPATITIS

(See Virus)

HIV

Ecological Formulas Monolaurin (600 mg capsules): 2 capsules
with meals—6 total

L-Lysine (1,000 mg tablets): 2 tablets per day on empty stomach

Ecological Formulas Nutricillin (capsules): 3 capsules per day with
food

Transfer Point Beta Glucan (500 mg capsules): 2 capsules per day
with food

Avoid processed sugars, fermented foods, egg yolks, nuts, dairy,
and red meat

HOT FLASHES

Homeopathic Sepia (pellets, 6X potency): dissolve 3 pellets under
tongue 3 times per day on empty stomach

Homeopathic Sulph Acidum (pellets, 6X potency): dissolve 3
pellets under tongue 3 times per day on empty stomach

Chasteberry (tincture): dissolve 25 drops in 3 ounces water 3
times per day on empty stomach

Evening Primrose Oil (300 mg capsules): 1 capsule per day on
empty stomach

HPV (HUMAN PAPILLOMA VIRUS)

(See HIV)

IMMUNITY

Solaray Propolis (500 mg capsules): 2 capsules per day on empty
stomach

Astragalus (tincture): dissolve 25 drops in 3 ounces water 3 times
per day on empty stomach

Vitamin C Complex (1,000 mg tablets): 2 tablets with meals—
6 total

IMPOTENCE

L-Arginine (500 mg capsules): 2 capsules 2 times per day on
empty stomach (omit if suffering from chronic virus)
Solaray Muira Puama (300 mg capsules): 2 capsules twice daily on
empty stomach
Vitamin E (Gamma) (400 units, capsules): 3 capsules per day on
empty stomach
Nature Most Zinc Gluconate (50 mg tablets): 1 tablet per day
with food

INFLUENZA

(See Virus)

INSOMNIA

Melatonin (3 mg tablets): 2 tablets before bed
Passion Flower (tincture): dissolve 25 drops in 3 ounces water
before bed
Natural Calm Magnesium Citrate (powder): 1 rounded teaspoon
in 4 ounces water before bed

JET LAG

Solaray Propolis (500 mg capsules): 2 capsules per day the day
before and the day of travel on empty stomach
Melatonin (3 mg tablets): 1 tablet the night before travel and
2 tablets the day of travel
Homeopathic No Jet Lag (pellets): as directed
Drink at least 60 ounces water per day for 1 week prior to and
during travel
Eat light meals for 48 hours prior to travel
Avoid caffeine and alcohol for 48 hours prior to and the day
of travel

JOINT HEALTH

Country Life MSM/GS Complex (tablets): 3 tablets per day with food

Boswellia (tincture): dissolve 25 drops in 3 ounces water 3 times per day on empty stomach

Natural Factors Celadrin (capsules): 3 capsules per day on empty stomach

KIDNEY STONES

(See Gallstones)

LIVER TOXICITY

Quantum Herbs Chaparral (tincture): dissolve 25 drops in 3 ounces water 3 times per day on empty stomach

Alpha Lipoic Acid (50 mg capsules): 2 capsules per day on empty stomach

Choline/Inositol (500 mg tablets): 2 tablets 2 times per day with food

Methionine (500 mg capsules): 2 capsules 2 times per day with food

L-Glutathione (500 mg capsules): 1 capsule 2 times per day on empty stomach

Lewis Labs Lecithin Granules: 3 tablespoons per day in beverage

LOU GEHRIG'S DISEASE (ALS)

Phosphatidyl Choline (300 mg capsules): 1 capsule with meals—3 total

Solgar Spirulina (750 mg tablets): 2 tablets with meals—6 per day

Nordic Naturals DHA (500 mg capsules): 2 capsules 2 times per day with food

EGCG Max (700 mg capsules): 2 capsules per day on empty
stomach

Now Grape Seed Extract (60 mg capsules): 2 capsules 2 times per
day with food

Jarrow Formulas B_{12} (Methylcobalamin) (5,000 mg tablets):
1 tablet per day with food

Standard Process Cataplex E (Pea Vine) (10 mg capsules):
1 capsule 2 times per day with food

LUNGS (OBSTRUCTED)

Mullein Tea: 3 cups per day

Myrrh (tincture): dissolve 25 drops in 3 ounces water 3 times per
day on empty stomach

L-Cysteine (500 mg capsules): 1 capsule 2 times per day on empty
stomach

Vitamin A (10,000 mg capsules): 1 per day on empty stomach

LUPUS

L-Cysteine (500 mg capsules): 1 capsule 2 times per day on empty
stomach

Solaray Propolis (500 mg capsules): 2 caps per day on empty
stomach

Solgar Spirulina (750 mg capsules): 2 capsules 3 times per day on
empty stomach

LYME DISEASE

Transfer Point Beta Glucan (500 mg capsules): 3 capsules per day
on empty stomach

Ecological Formulas Nutricillin (capsules): 3 capsules per day with
food

Enzymatic Therapy Saventaro (Cat's Claw) (20 mg capsules):
2 capsules per day on empty stomach

Arrow Formulas Resist-Immune (capsules): 2 capsules per day on empty stomach

Vitamin C Complex (1,000 mg capsules): 2 capsules with meals—6 total

Oreganol Oil (drops): dissolve 10 drops in 3 ounces water 3 times per day

Avoid fermented food and nuts

LYMPHATIC INFLAMMATION

Red Clover Tea: 3 cups per day

Clove (tincture): dissolve 10 drops in 3 ounces water 3 times per day on empty stomach

Pantothenic Acid (500 mg capsules): 1 capsule with meals—3 total

MACULAR DEGENERATION

(See Glaucoma)

MENINGITIS

(See Virus)

MENSTRUAL BLEEDING (DELAYED)/AMENORRHEA

Fennel Seed/Sesame Seed/Cumin Seed Tea (3-seed tea): 3 cups per day

Now Grape Seed Extract (60 mg capsules): 3 capsules 2 times per day on empty stomach

MENSTRUAL BLEEDING (EXCESSIVELY HEAVY)

Homeopathic Arnica (pellets, 6X potency): dissolve 3 pellets under tongue 3 times per day on empty stomach

Lady's Mantle (tincture): dissolve 25 drops in 3 ounces water 3 times per day on empty stomach

Solgar Hemantic (tablets): 1 tablet with meals—3 total

Eliminate caffeine, alcohol, tobacco, and spicy foods

MENSTRUAL CRAMPS

Motherwort (tincture): dissolve 25 drops in 3 ounces water
3 times per day on empty stomach

DL-Phenylalanine (500 mg tablets): 1 tablet 3 times per day on
empty stomach

Homeopathic Hypericum (pellets, 30c potency): dissolve 3 pellets
under tongue 3 times per day on empty stomach

Serrapeptase (20,000 units, capsules): 1 capsule 3 times per day
on empty stomach

MOLD ALLERGIES

BioAllers Mold, Yeast & Dust (tincture): dissolve 6 drops under
tongue 3 times per day on empty stomach

Grapefruit Seed Extract (drops): dissolve 6 drops in 3 ounces
water 3 times per day with food

Solgar Caprylic Acid (tablets): 1 tablet with meals—3 total

Vitamin C Complex (1,000 mg tablets): 2 tablets with meals—
6 total

MOOD SWINGS

Bach Flower Remedies Hornbeam (drops): dissolve 3 drops in
3 ounces water 3 times per day

Homeopathic Ignatia (pellets, 30c potency): dissolve 3 pellets
under tongue 3 times per day on empty stomach

Chromium (200 mcg tablets): 1 tablet with meals—3 total

B complex (100 mg tablets): 1 tablet with meals—3 total

Nordic Naturals DHA (500 mg capsules): 1 with meals—
3 total

MORNING SICKNESS

Ginger (500 mg capsules): 2 capsules 2 times per day on empty
stomach

Black Horehound Tea: 2 cups per day on empty stomach
PSI Brand Acupressure Bands: as directed

MOTION SICKNESS

Homeopathic Lac Defloratum (pellets, 6X potency): dissolve
    3 pellets under tongue 3 times per day on empty stomach

MULTIPLE SCLEROSIS

(See Lou Gehrig's Disease)

NAIL FUNGUS

Baking soda and hydrogen peroxide (prepare a paste): apply
    morning and evening for 4 months
(See Candidiasis)

NAUSEA

Homeopathic Ipecac (pellets, 30X potency): dissolve 3 pellets
    under tongue 3 times per day on empty stomach
Ginger Tea: 1 cup 3 times per day

NERVE PAIN

Homeopathic Hypericum (pellets, 30c potency): dissolve 3 pellets
    under tongue 3 times per day on empty stomach
Nordic Naturals Omega 3 Fish Oil (capsules): 2 capsules 2 times
    per day with food

OSTEOPOROSIS

(See Acidosis and Bone Health)

PANCREATITIS

Nature Most Multi Enzyme (tablets): 1 tablet at breakfast and
    lunch only

L-Methionine (500 mg capsules): 1 capsule 2 times per day on
   empty stomach
L-Glutamine (500 mg capsules): 1 capsule 2 times per day on
   empty stomach
Biotics Nutriclear Meal Replacement (powder): blend
   2 tablespoons with 10 ounces rice milk at
   breakfast
Test for food reactions
Avoid alcohol, caffeine, and tobacco

PARASITES (THREE-WEEK PROTOCOL)

Black Walnut (tincture): dissolve 10 drops in 3 ounces water
   2 times per day
Wormwood (tincture): dissolve 25 drops in 3 ounces water 3 times
   per day on empty stomach
Pumpkin Seeds: ¼ cup 2 times per day

PARKINSON'S DISEASE

(See Lou Gehrig's Disease)

PMS

Vitamin B$_6$ 100 (100 mg tablets): 1 tablet with meals—3 total
Vitamin E (Gamma) (400 units, capsules): 1 capsule 2 times per
   day with food
DIM (100 mg tablets): 1 tablet on empty stomach
Kava Kava (tincture): dissolve 25 drops in 3 ounces water 3 times
   per day on empty stomach

PNEUMONIA

(See Virus; Immunity)

POISON IVY

Homeopathic Rhus Tox (pellets, 6X potency): dissolve 3 pellets under tongue 3 times per day on empty stomach

Jewelweed (spray): apply topically as directed by day

Calendula (cream): apply topically as directed before bed

PROGESTERONE (DEFICIENCY)

Alvia Progensa Transdermal Bio Identical Progesterone (cream): rub ¼ teaspoon on wrists before bed every other night

Wild Yam (200 mg capsules): 1 capsule 2 times per day on empty stomach

PROSTATITIS (BENIGN PROSTATE HYPERTROPHY)

Homeopathic Sabal Serrulata (pellets, 30X potency): dissolve 3 pellets under tongue 3 times per day on empty stomach

Nature's Way Pygeum (50 mg capsules): 1 capsule 3 times per day on empty stomach

Quercetin Plus (Kurt Donsbach Prostasol) (capsules): 1 capsule per day on empty stomach

Nature's Most Zinc Gluconate (50 mg tablets): 1 tablet per day with food

PSORIASIS

(See Eczema)

SARCOIDOSIS

Serrapeptase (20,000 units, capsules): 1 capsule 3 times per day on empty stomach

Bromelain (500 mg capsules): 1 capsule 3 times per day on empty stomach

Turmeric Root (500 mg capsules): 2 capsules 2 times per day on empty stomach

Nordic Naturals Ultimate Omega (liquid): 1 tablespoon 3 times
    per day with food
Rosemary (500 mg capsules): 2 capsules 2 times per day on empty
    stomach

SEIZURES
(See Epilepsy)

SINUS INFLAMMATION (CHRONIC)
Chrysanthemum Flower Tea: 3 cups per day
Clove (tincture): dissolve 10 drops in 3 ounces water 3 times
    per day
Homeopathic Kali Bichromicum (pellets, 6X potency): dissolve
    3 pellets under tongue 3 times per day on empty stomach
Neti Pot (with sea salt): follow neti pot directions

SLEEP DISORDERS
(See Insomnia)

SPIDER VEINS
Homeopathic Hamamelis Virginicus (pellets, 6X potency):
    dissolve 3 pellets under tongue 3 times per day on empty
    stomach
Bioflavonoid Complex (500 mg tablets): 2 tablets 2 times per day
    with food

THYROID (HYPER)
Lemon Balm (tincture): dissolve 25 drops in 3 ounces water
    3 times per day on empty stomach
Natural Calm Magnesium Citrate (powder): dissolve 1 rounded
    teaspoon in 4 ounces water 3 times per day
L-Glutamine (500 mg capsules): 1 capsule 2 times per day on
    empty stomach

Rosemary (500 mg capsules): 2 capsules 2 times per day on empty
stomach

Turmeric Root (500 mg capsules): 2 capsules 2 times per day on
empty stomach

THYROID (HYPO)

Selenium (200 mcg capsules): 1 capsule per day with food

Nature Most Zinc Gluconate (50 mg tablets): 1 tablet per day
with food

Kelp (250 mcg tablets): 1 tablet every other day

L-Tyrosine (500 mg capsules): 1 capsule 2 times per day on empty
stomach

Pyridoxyl-5-Phosphate (50 mg capsules): 1 capsule 2 times per
day with food

TINNITUS (RINGING IN EARS)

Twin Labs Potassium Citrate (liquid): 1 teaspoon per day with
food

Natural Calm Magnesium Citrate (powder): 2 teaspoons per day
in water

ULCER (DIGESTIVE TRACT)

German Chamomile Tea: 3 cups per day served at room
temperature

ProFibe Fruit Pectin (powder): 1 scoop 3 times per day in water
between meals

Biotics NutriClear Meal Replacement (rice) (powder): 2 scoops
blended with 10 ounces rice milk at breakfast

16 ounces freshly made cabbage and pear juice per day

VERTIGO (DIZZINESS)

(See Tinnitus)

VIRUS

Transfer Point Beta Glucan (500 mg capsules): 2 capsules per day
  with food

Ecological Formulas Nutricillin (capsules): 3 capsules per day with
  food

Ecological Formulas Monolaurin (600 mg capsules): 2 capsules
  with meals—6 total

Lemon Balm (tincture): dissolve 25 drops in 3 ounces water
  3 times per day on empty stomach

L-Lysine (1,000 mg tablets): 2 tablets per day on empty stomach

Umcka (syrup): as directed

Avoid processed sugars, fermented foods, egg yolks, nuts, dairy,
  and red meat

WARTS

Tea Tree Oil and Swedish Bitters: topically apply equal parts with
  Q-Tip, 1 time morning and 1 time evening for 2 weeks

APPENDIX B
EMT Long Form Chart

ELECTROMAGNETIC MUSCLE TESTING (EMT)
Body Assessment

VITAL ORGAN	ENERGY PULSE RATING	CAUSAL ROOT				
		DIET	MENTAL	EMOTIONAL	CHEMICAL	STRUCTURAL
LIVER						
GALLBLADDER						
HEART						
SMALL INTESTINE						
SPLEEN						
STOMACH						
LUNGS						
LARGE INTESTINE						
KIDNEYS						
BLADDER						
GLANDS						
ADRENAL CORTEX						
ADRENAL MEDULLA						
THYROID						
PARATHYROID						
THYMUS						
PANCREAS						
THALAMUS						
HYPOTHALAMUS						
OVARIES						
MAMMARIES						
TESTES						
PROSTATE						
PINEAL						
PITUITARY						

ADDITIONAL

BACTERIAL _____ STAPH _____ MOLD _____ STREP _____ CRANIAL YEAST _____

SACRAL YEAST _____ INFECTIOUS VIRUS _____ RETROVIRUS _____

GLAND/ORGAN ROOT REFERENCE _____

ELECTROMAGNETIC MUSCLE TESTING (EMT)
Brain Assessment

CEREBRAL CORTEX

Right Prefrontal Cortex (protective emotional memory) _____

Left Prefrontal Cortex (confidence and reasoning) _____

Corpus Callosum (bridge that balances left and right) _____

Parietal Lobe (movement) _____

Occipital Lobe (visual perception) _____

Temporal Lobe (auditory perception) _____

LIMBIC SYSTEM

Hippocampus (protective emotional memory) _____

Amygdala (protective emotional memory) _____

CEREBELLUM

Cerebral Cortex (balance and coordination) _____

BRAIN STEM

Midbrain (spinal-brain relay) _____

Pons (organ motor system) _____

Medulla Oblongata (sleep and arousal) _____

ELECTROMAGNETIC MUSCLE TESTING (EMT)
Mind Assessment

1. *Conscious Mind (12 percent of brain capacity)—present moment reasoning and decisions* _____

2. *Unconscious/Subconscious Mind (88 percent of brain capacity)—stores all life events* _____

3. *Ego/Conditioned Mind (identifies with material reality)* _____

4. *Id (seeks to satisfy physical needs)* _____

5. *Superego (conscience/self-critic)* _____

6. *Superconscious Mind/Soul (the observer/source consciousness)* _____

APPENDIX C
EMT Food Chart

● Alkaline Foods　　□ Neutral Foods　　● Acid Foods

ANIMAL PROTEIN
beef ●
chicken ●
clam ●
cod ●
crab ●
egg white ●
egg yolk ●
flounder ●
haddock ●
halibut ●
ham ●
lamb ●
liver ●
lobster ●
pork ●
salmon ●
sardine ●
scallop ●
shrimp ●
sole ●
tuna ●
turkey ●

DAIRY, DAIRY SUBSTITUTES
almond milk ●
cow's cheese ●
cow's milk □
cow's yogurt □
rice milk ●
rice milk cheese ●
soy cheese ●
soy milk ●
soy yogurt ●

BEANS
adzuki ●
anasaki ●
black ●
chickpea ●
kidney ●
lentil ●
mung ●
navy ●
northern ●
pinto ●
soy/tofu ●
white ●

NUTS/SEEDS
almond ●
Brazil ●
cashew ●
macadamia ●
peanut ●
pecan ●
pine ●
pistachio ●
pumpkin ●
sesame ●
sunflower ●
walnut ●

FATS
avocado ●
butter ●
coconut ●
cream ●
ghee ●
margarine ●
vegetable oil □

LOW-STARCH VEGETABLES
arugula ●
asparagus ●
broccoli ●
Brussels sprouts ●
cabbage ●
cauliflower ●
celery ●
Chinese cabbage ●
collard ●
cucumber ●
eggplant ●
endive ●
escarole ●
garlic ●
green beans ●
kale ●
kohlrabi ●
leek ●
lettuce ●
lotus root ●
mushroom ●
mustard green ●
okra ●
onion ●
parsley ●
pepper ●
radish ●
scallion ●
sorrel ●
spinach ●
sprouts ●
summer squash ●
Swiss chard ●
turnip ●
turnip green ●
watercress ●
zucchini ●

HIGH-STARCH VEGETABLES
artichoke ●
beet ●
carrot ●
chestnut ●
corn ●
lima bean ●
parsnip ●
pea ●
potato ●
pumpkin ●
winter squash ●
yam ●

GRAIN PRODUCTS (STARCH)
amaranth ●
barley ●
buckwheat ●
kamut ●
kasha ●
millet ●
oats ●
quinoa ●
rice ●
rye ●
spelt ●
triticale ●
wheat ●

SUGARS
barley malt ●
brown sugar ●
honey ●
maple syrup ●
rice syrup ●
sucanat ●
stevia ●
turbinado ●
white bread ●
white sugar ●

ACID FRUITS
grapefruit ◆
kiwi ◆
kumquat ◆
lemon ◆
lime ◆
orange ◆
pineapple ◆
strawberry ◆
tomato ◆

SUB ACID FRUITS
apple ●
apricot ●
blackberry ●
blueberry ●
cherry ●
grape ●
mango ●
nectarine ●
papaya ●
peach ●
pear ●
plum ●
raspberry ●
tangerine ●

SWEET FRUITS
banana ●
currant ●
date ●
fig ●
raisin ●

MELONS
cantaloupe ●
casaba ●
Christmas ●
honeydew ●
musk ●
watermelon ●

MISC.
fruit preserve ●
sugar-free jam ●
vinegar ●

Key
● Alkaline Foods—eat 4 for each 1 acid food
● Acid Foods—eat 1 for each 4 alkaline foods
□ Neutral Foods—remain neutral only when your pH is stable
◆ Acid Foods that convert to alkaline only when your pH is stable

APPENDIX D

EMT PERSONALIZED MANTRA ASSESSMENT

VOWEL TEST

A

E

I

O

U

MUSICAL KEY TEST

A

B

C

D

E

F

G

TEST RESULTS

Number of days per week mantra exercise performed:

Duration of mantra session:

Optimal time of day:

Should protocol be changed at some point, and if so, how?:

Relative power of personalized mantra:

APPENDIX E
Illustrated Shen Clearing Chart

The Five Negative Zhang and Fu Emotions: Scale: Minus 1–10

1. Anger (Lv)
2. Hatred (Ht)
3. Anxiety (Sp)
4. Grief (Lu)
5. Fear (Kd)

Internal Root Reference: Scale: Minus 1–10

1. Mother
2. Father
3. Natal family
4. Married family
5. Culture
6. World
7. Self

Ages of Shen Blockages

1	21	41	61
2	22	42	62
3	23	43	63
4	24	44	64
5	25	45	65
6	26	46	66
7	27	47	67
8	28	48	68
9	29	49	69
10	30	50	70
11	31	51	71
12	32	52	72
13	33	53	73
14	34	54	74
15	35	55	75
16	36	56	76
17	37	57	77
18	38	53	78
19	39	59	79
20	40	60	80

Each of the above Shen blockages should be pulse tested from minus 1 to 10

ACKNOWLEDGMENTS

I'd like to express my appreciation to Monique Parent for her illustrations, Vanessa Mincolla for polishing and editing, Nick Mincolla for polishing and editing, Joel Price for technical editing, Lex Mincolla for consulting support, Amie Theriault for text formatting and technical assistance, Kerry Brett for cover portrait photography, and Andrew Yackira and Joel Fotinos for their continued support.

INDEX